药理学自主实验设计与典型案例参考

Independent Design of the Pharmacology Experiment & Typical Case Study

主　编　徐卫东　魏　渊

主　审　高　静

副主编　李　静　孙　竞

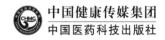

中国健康传媒集团
中国医药科技出版社

内容提要

本教材紧扣药学留学生教学大纲和培养细则。近年来，在国内外建立的药师工作以"物"为中心的发药型，向"以病人为中心"的药学服务型工作模式转变，据此全书内容共分三个模块，分别介绍了基础药理学实验、临床药理学实验和药学服务指导，具有较强的针对性，同时突出药理学实验技能与应用能力的培养。

本教材围绕药学留学生需要掌握的各种实验、实践专业知识和技能展开阐述，专业性强，可供从事药学与相关领域人员参考。

图书在版编目（CIP）数据

药理学自主实验设计与典型案例参考 = Independent Design of the Pharmacology Experiment & Typical Case Study：汉、英 / 徐卫东，魏渊主编 .—北京：中国医药科技出版社，2022.11

ISBN 978-7-5214-3470-5

Ⅰ.①药… Ⅱ.①徐… ②魏… Ⅲ.①药理学—实验—高等学校—教学参考资料—汉、英 Ⅳ.① R965.2

中国版本图书馆 CIP 数据核字（2022）第 197688 号

美术编辑 陈君杞
责任编辑 吴思思 张 睿
版式设计 友全图文

出版 **中国健康传媒集团** | 中国医药科技出版社
地址 北京市海淀区文慧园北路甲 22 号
邮编 100082
电话 发行：010-62227427 邮购：010-62236938
网址 www.cmstp.com
规格 787×1092mm $^1/_{16}$
印张 14 $^3/_4$
字数 320 千字
版次 2022 年 11 月第 1 版
印次 2022 年 11 月第 1 次印刷
印刷 三河市万龙印装有限公司
经销 全国各地新华书店
书号 ISBN 978-7-5214-3470-5
定价 **60.00 元**

获取新书信息、投稿、为图书纠错，请扫码联系我们。

编 委 会

主　编　徐卫东　魏　渊

主　审　高　静

副主编　李　静　孙　竞

编　者（以姓氏笔画为序）

王治平（广东药科大学）

孙　竞（江苏大学药学院）

孙全才（新加坡国立大学）

李　静（江苏大学药学院）

张逸帆（伦敦国王学院）

郑　义（山东大学药学院）

闻　艺（郑州大学医学院）

钱元霞（镇江市第二人民医院）

徐卫东（江苏大学药学院）

彭　晔（澳门科技大学医学院）

魏　渊（江苏大学药学院）

绘　图　张思皖（中央美术学院造型学院）

Preface

Scientific innovations significantly accelerate the development of social economy, especially in the pharmaceutical industry. Pharmacology experiment, a compulsory course of the national top undergraduate major in our school, plays an important role in training creative thinking, inspiring drug design, strengthening life science knowledge and experimental skills, and building Chinese core socialist values for students.

Since the former teaching framework of this course was relatively weak in supporting independent experiment design, striving to achieve the training object of 'mastering knowledge, good at research, open-minded and skilled in industry production', we reconfigured the teaching module and greatly increased the case of independent study design in this textbook to train the innovative ability of students, supported by multi-media and flipped class model.

This textbook mainly consists of three parts below to help students master both the theory and practical skills. Firstly, to train basic study skills of students with classical experiment cases, helping them learn to use common laboratory equipment and initially cultivate observation and practical research ability. In the second part, independent pharmacology experiment cases would encourage the student to optimize their study design by collecting and reading literature materials, and analyze their experiment results via oral defense. Last but not least, we provide relevant guidelines that students should follow when participating in community pharmacy practice.

As one of the important explorations of innovation-oriented pharmacology teaching reform, this textbook also made a significant innovation in the compilation method. We provided English-based contents and Chinese translations to help readers get more familiar with pharmaceutical vocabulary and facilitate international students' learning. However, limited by our academic and writing level, there might be some mistakes in this book. It would be greatly appreciated if you could provide any constructive feedback and corrections.

Editor

2022.8

前　言

　　坚持以"科技创新"为动力，充分激发"创新创造"活力是实现社会经济高质量发展的重要战略之一。作为国民经济的重要组成部分，医药产业的"科创"发展至关重要。药理学实验作为江苏大学药学院国家一流专业必修课程，在帮助药学专业本科生树立社会主义核心价值观，巩固药学、基础医学和生命科学核心理论和实验技能，启迪新药研发和创新思维等方面发挥重要作用。

　　原先的药理学实验教学方案框架较为固定、对学生参与自主试验设计的支撑度相对不足，本教材以培养学生药学"科创"能力为目标导向、坚持"三全育人"思想，重构实验教学内容模块、大幅增加学生自主实验设计案例，并与教学中"新媒体互动理论教学"和"翻转课堂讨论"深度呼应，力求实现"精理论、擅研究、新视野、晓生产"培养目标定位。

　　本教材按照以上理念将药理实验学习划分为以下几个部分：第一部分为基础技能培养，通过一些经典实验理论知识学习，帮助学生学会使用常见实验仪器和设备，初步培养学生的实际操作能力和实验观察能力；第二部分为自主药理学实验案例参考，鼓励学生搜集文献资料以优化实验方案，并对预期结果进行分析与答辩；第三部分为药学服务，制定了学生参与医疗实践环节中应该遵循的相关指南。通过上述三个部分的学习，帮助学生储备扎实的药理学实验理论和提高实验操作技能。

　　作为"科创"导向性药理学的教学改革重要探索内容之一，本教材也在编写方式上做出了重要创新，即采用英文为主、汉语对照编写方式，帮助学生进一步熟悉药学专业英语并方便药学专业留学生参与实验学习。限于编者的学术与编写水平，本教材难免存在一些不足，恳请广大读者批评指正。

编　者

2022 年 8 月

目 录
Catalogue

Chapter 1　Basic Theories in Pharmacology Experiment

第一篇　药理学实验基础知识

Chapter 2   Typical Cases of Independent Experimental Design in Basic Pharmacology

第二篇 基础药理学自主实验设计典型案例

Chapter 3　Basic Clinical Pharmacology Experiments

第三篇　基础临床药理学自主实验设计典型案例

Chapter 4　Clinical Pharmacology Practice

第四篇　临床药理学实习

Introduction

Knowledge

1. The objective and significance of the pharmacology experiment course.
2. The content and format of experimental report writing.
3. The collation requirements of experimental results.
4. Three stages in studying pharmacology experiments.
5. The significance of original records and collation of experimental results.

Skill

The basic knowledge and ability required of independent experimental skills in pharmacology.

Three Stages in Studying Pharmacology Experiments

Pharmacology is a practical subject that requires a great number of experiments for better understanding. The level of pharmacology experiment skill directly affects the capability of drug research. This pharmacology experiment course offers students a chance to discover the effect of drugs on your own, to enhance your understanding and ability in pharmacology. Pharmacology experiments can also benefit the student in further studies by training your experiments skills, including observation, comparison, analysis, summarising and solving real-world tasks.

Commonly, there are three stages in learning pharmacology experiments.

Stage 1: basic experiments and lab skills.

In this stage, you will study how to use lab equipments, then review and verify the knowledge you have learnt in a series of classic experiments.

Stage 2: comprehensive experiments and skills of solving complex tasks.

Carry out pharmacology experiments based on knowledge from anatomy, physiology, pathophysiology and other subjects.

Stage 3: independent pharmacology experiments and training research ability.

1. Independently design pharmacology experiments based on your own knowledge and

reliable references.

2. Defense your experiment design, including its background, objectives, methods and expected results with your teacher and other students.

3. Optimise the study design and put it into practice.

Objectives of the Pharmacology Experiment Course

1. Study the Methodology of Pharmaceutical Science

1.1 Theoretical findings come from the practice.

1.2 Review and verify theoretical knowledge in practice.

1.3 Understand the relevance among physiology, pathophysiology and other subjects, then systematically understand the human body and disease.

1.4 Have scientific observation, independent and cooperative study ability, and a serious attitude in experiments.

2. Train Basic Lab Skills

2.1 Induce disease models on lab animals, and practise basic lab skills.

2.2 Truthfully record and analyse the experiment result.

2.3 Finish experiment reports and improve your ability of writing research paper.

3. Improve the Research Ability

3.1 Train your research ability by comprehensive experiments and independent studies.

3.2 Learn the method of pre-clinical pharmacology studies for further subjects.

Requirements of the Course

1. Preview the experiment, especially in terms of its objectives, methods, process and required lab skills.

2. Prepare equipments and drugs, then double-check them before use.

3. Teamwork.

4. Carefully observe the experiment and truthfully record its result.

5. Compliance with laboratory regulations, including safety first, keep quiet, clean the lab after the experiment, etc.

6. Collate experiment results and finish study reports.

Data from pharmacology experiments are either quantitative, such as blood pressure and heart rate, or qualitative, including death count and survival. Analyse these results from the whole class if necessary with charts and statistical methods, then compose the experiment report.

Requirements of Writing Experiment Reports

As an essential skill in pharmaceutical study, composing experiment report benefits logical thinking and comprehensive analysis, and is in favour of writing paper in the future. Those reports should be neat and logical with a complete structure.

Besides name, student ID, date and location of the experiment, those contents below should be covered in the experiment report:

1. Title of the experiment: briefly describe the experiment based on its purpose.

2. Objectives: the aim of the experiment, not requirements of this course.

3. Methods: briefly describe the process of this experiment, focus on lab animals, drugs and administrations, and how to observe the phenomenon and record the result in the study. Do not just copy the tutorial.

4. Results: a core content of experiment reports.

Truthfully state the experiment results, with charts or tables if necessary, after the data management. You should also describe your findings in this part.

5. Discussion: another core content of experiment reports.

Analyse the study result, especially those unexpected ones, based on your theoretical knowledge.

6. Conclusion: briefly summarise the study result based on its objectives.

7. Reference: list the reference if necessary, and be aware of its format.

Appendix: Requirements of Original Experiment Records

Original experiment records are the first hand data of pharmaceutical studies and must be recorded accurately and clearly without alternation. With those original data, researchers in the future could rebuild the study. Meanwhile, original experiment record is also a significant part of Good Laboratory Practice (GLP).

Original experiment records of the experiment should contain the date, methods, staffs, findings, notes, etc. Photos and other printed materials are also acceptable in these records. Any alternation, if necessary, must not cover or blur the original record. A mark, signature and the reason are required when alternate the record.

Hand in the original experiment record, along with your study report.

绪 论

知识要求

1. 掌握药理学实验目的、意义。

2. 掌握实验报告撰写内容及格式。

3. 熟悉实验结果的整理要求。

4. 了解药理学实验学习的三大阶段。

5. 了解原始记录及实验结果整理的意义。

能力要求

了解药理学自主实验技能培养所需的基本知识和素质能力。

一、药理学实验学习的三大阶段

药理学是一门实验性科学。药理实验水平的优劣直接影响了未来新药研究能力的高低。开设药理实验课可以为学生还原药物效应发现时的原始场景，提高学生对药理学概念的感性认识，加深对相关药理学理论知识的理解水平。通过药理学实验还可以培养学生的实验操作能力和对实验对象观察、比较、分析、综合和解决实际问题的能力，帮助学生掌握一定的药理实验技能，为后续课程的学习打下基础。

药理实验学习可以分为以下三个阶段：第一阶段为基础技能培养，通过一些经典实验，验证和巩固理论知识，学会使用常用仪器设备，初步培养学生的实际操作能力和实验观察能力；第二阶段为综合性实验实训，该阶段将解剖学、生理学、病理生理学、药理学的理论知识有机融合，培养学生综合分析问题能力和科研能力；第三阶段为自主药理学实验，要求学生通过查阅文献资料，撰写实验方案，并对设计方案的背景知识、实验目的、实验方法、预期结果进行设计答辩。由教师和学生提出问题后，对实验的技术路线和实行方案做出切合实际的修改，再由学生自行完成实验。通过上述三个阶段的训练，可为学生以后的科研工作奠定坚实的理论和实验操作基础。

二、药理学实验课的目的

（一）培养科学的观点

1.培养学生理论来自实验的观点。

2.加深、验证和巩固理论知识，培养学生理论联系实际的能力。

3.综合应用生理学、药理学、病理生理学等学科的相关知识和实验方法，使学生初步建立整体、全面、系统的人体观和疾病观。

4.培养学生勤于动手、善于观察、科学分析和独立工作的能力，养成对科学工作的严肃态度，以及严格要求、严谨工作、团结协作和实事求是的工作作风。

（二）训练基本实验技能

1.学习在动物身上复制典型病理过程和人类疾病的基本实验方法和原理，掌握功能试验常用的仪器设备和基本技术。

2.通过书写原始记录，培养学生捕捉实验现象的技能和严谨诚实的科研态度。

3.通过书写实验报告，培养学生科研论文的写作能力。

（三）培养学生科学研究的能力及综合分析问题的能力

1.通过综合性实验和学生自主设计实验，培养学生科研工作的能力。

2.通过学习新药临床前药理学研究方法，为从事新药的药理学、毒理学研究打下基础。

三、实验课的要求

1. **预习**　仔细阅读所要进行的实验内容，结合所学理论，认真领会实验目的和原理，熟悉操作方法与步骤，并对实验结果进行理论推测，做到心中有数。

2. **清点药品和器材**　实验操作前对照实验教程检查药品名称和浓度、器材数量和性能，安排好药品和器材的摆放位置，以防错拿错放。

3. **合理分工和正确操作**　每个实验小组在实验过程中要合理分工，互相配合完成实验，包括调试仪器、动物手术、药量换算、给药方法等都要做到准确无误。

4. **认真观察和记录**　实验时要仔细观察实验现象，如动物用药后的反应差异、反应持续时间及转归，并如实记录在原始记录本上，不许随意涂改。

5. **遵守实验室规则**　安全操作，防止触电、药物中毒、动物咬伤等事故，实验过程中必须保持实验室安静。实验结束后，要将所用器材擦洗干净并放回指定位置；检查仪器性能，填写使用记录，如有损坏要报告带教老师，并进行登记。实验动物按要求处理，安排值日，打扫实验室卫生。

6. **整理实验资料、书写实验报告**　药理实验资料可分为量反应资料（如血压、心率、平滑肌收缩幅度等）和质反应资料（如动物死亡与存活数）。将实验资料加以整理，如通过设计图、表格进行比较分析，或进行统计学处理（必要时，综合全班实验资料），按要求写出实验报告。

四、实验报告的撰写要求

书写实验报告是实验研究工作的基本功之一，有助于提高逻辑思维和综合分析能力，也可为撰写研究论文打下基础。实验报告要求文字简练切题，书写工整，结构完整，项目齐全，注意科学性和逻辑性。

实验报告除一般项目（姓名、学号、时间、地点等）外，应包括如下内容：

（1）**实验题目**　根据实验研究目的，简明扼要写出实验题目。

（2）**实验目的**　只要求写实验研究目的，不必写实验原理及实验课的要求。

（3）**实验方法**　宜用简练的文字写明实验大体操作步骤，着重说明所用动物或标本、药品及器材、给药剂量及途径、如何观察及记录实验结果等，切忌抄写实验教程。

（4）**实验结果**　将原始记录本上实验所得数据整理并统计处理后，如实表述，或以图形、表格形式表述。此部分为实验报告的重点内容，数据结果必须经统计分析处理，不可将原始记录照搬于实验报告中。除了数据处理外，实验结果还包括对实验现象及对实验结果的文字描述，要求描述客观，准确。

（5）**讨论**　此部分内容亦为实验报告的重点。讨论应针对实验中观察到的现象和结果进行分析推理，逐步推导出结论，切不可离开实验结果而空谈理论。实验中如得不到预期结果或与其他组实验结果不一致，则应仔细分析其原因。

（6）结论　实验结论是从实验结果归纳而得到的概括性判断，应与实验目的相对应，文字应简练、明确、严谨，不可超出本实验结果所说明的问题。

（7）参考文献　实验报告书写过程中参考的文献均可列于实验报告后，注意书写格式正确。

附：实验原始记录要求

实验原始资料是实验结果的第一手资料，任何一项实验研究的原始资料都必须清楚、正确、不加涂改地记录在册。由此得出的实验研究报告和结论，若干年后在没有有关人员的情况下仍可以单独从这些数据中重新建立。实验原始资料也是实验室质量管理规范（Good Laboratory Practice，GLP）的主要内容之一。实验原始记录包括：实验日期、实验方法、实验人员的分工、实验研究过程中各种实验现象的观察、备忘录和注释，还可以包括照片、计算机打印材料和自动设备记录的材料等。对记录的任何变更都不得覆盖原有的记录或使其看不清楚，应该用单线划标记，然后写上变更的内容，说明变更的原因并签名。实验结束后，随实验报告一并上交带教老师批阅。

第一篇
药理学实验基础知识

Chapter 1

Basic Theories in Pharmacology Experiment

Section 1　Basic Theories in Experiment Animals

~ . ~ . ~ . ~ . ~ . ~ . ~ . ~ . ~ . ~ . ~ . ~ . ~ .

Knowledge

1. Basic requirements of selecting lab animals.

2. Features of common experiment animals.

3. Classification and applications of experiment animals.

Skill

Rationally select lab animals based on the study purpose.

~ . ~ . ~ . ~ . ~ . ~ . ~ . ~ . ~ . ~ . ~ . ~ . ~ .

Requirements for Experiment Animals

We mainly conduct animals as study objects in pharmacology experiments. It is very important to select suitable lab animals for better reliability and accuracy of the study.

Lab animals are classified into 4 grades according to their microbiological control standards:

1. Conventional Animals (CVs)

Generally, CVs carry no zoonotic diseases or severe infectious diseases.

2. Clean Animals (CLs)

CLs are more controlled than CVs, as they do not carry pathogens that are harmful to animals or those may interfere the experiment. This is the basic level of lab animals in scientific research.

3. Specific Pathogen Free Animals (SPFs)

SPFs are even more controlled than CLs. They do not carry a list of specific micro-organisms and parasites.

4. Germ Free Animals (GFs) & Gnotobiotic Animals (GNs)

There is no detectable micro-organisms and parasites inside or outside the GF.

GNs are GFs that got implanted with some specific micro-organisms or parasites.

Besides the feature of lab animals and the experience of inducing disease models on specific animals, we should also consider these questions as follows when select lab animals: whether and how likely can the disease model be successfully replicated, if the observation is feasible, how stable the method is, and the cost of the study, etc.

Select Experiment Animals

Commonly-used mammal animals in pharmacology experiments are listed as follows: mice, rats, guinea pigs, rabbits, dogs, cats, and monkeys. All of them have some similar physiological features to human.

A brief introduction of those animals is listed below.

1. Toads and Frogs

Toads and frogs are easy to raise. As their isolated hearts can still beat for a relatively long period, they are often applied in cardiac insufficiency and pathogenic heart models. Furthermore, their sciatic nerve and gastrocnemius muscle are usually used in observing drug effects, especially local anaesthetics and muscle relaxants, on peripheral nerves, neuromuscular junctions or striated muscles. Besides, frog tongues and their mesenteries are ideal specimens for observing inflammation and the change of microcirculation. In addition, we may also carry out experiments to study edema and renal insufficiency on frogs.

2. Mice

Mice are easy to reproduce, hence they are suitable for experiments that require a great number of animals, such as determining the median lethal dose and preliminary drug screenings. They have a very strong reproductive ability, with a only-20-day gestation period.

We can replicate many pathological models on mice, such as edema, inflammation, hypoxia, various tumours, etc. They can also be employed in screening contraceptives and anti-tumour drugs, and carcinogenicity studies.

Compared with other lab animals, mice models have these features below:

2.1 Mice are the most commonly-used lab animal. They are very cheap and easy to reproduce, and can easily meet the requirement of species, gender and age. Besides, mice do not require strict living conditions.Hence, mouse models are always utilised when meet the experiment requirement.

2.2 Mice are susceptible to many diseases, therefore they are suitable for studying these illnesses, such as schistosomiasis, malaria, influenza, encephalitis, etc. Mice have lots of pure-breed strains, some of them have unique features and are susceptible to some certain diseases. For example, C3HA mice are sensitive to cancer, whereas C57 mice are'anti-cancer'. Hence, mice models are widely employed in tumour researches.

2.3 Mice organs are small and easy to observe, therefore they are very suitable for studies using electron microscope, in order to save cost. For example, observe chronic bronchitis lungs.

2.4 Mice have developed nerve system and can be used to replicate neurosis models.

2.5 Mice have poor adaptability to the environment, such as inappropriate temperature and lack of food. Therefore, be patient, careful and gently in mouse experiments.

3. Rats

Rats are similar to mice, but larger. We can also replicate pathological models on rats, including edema, inflammation, hypoxia, shock, etc. Compared with other lab animals, rat models have these features below:

3.1 Rats are also easy to reproduce and raise, hence they are suitable for experiments that require a large amount of animals when mice do not meet the study requirement. For example, oral and parenteral administrations of nitrosamine can cause esophageal cancer in rats, but not in mice. Therefore we choose rats in such studies.

3.2 Rats are larger than mice, therefore they are more suitable than mice in experiments that require larger bodies. For example, we can directly read their blood pressure, and they have more sensitive blood pressure response than the rabbit. Rats can be used to study the change of blood circulation during shock and disseminated intravascular coagulation (DIC). Their hindlimb can be employed in limb vascular perfusion experiments. Furthermore, the isolated heart of rats can also be applied in experiments. Moreover, we may collect the lymph from rats' thoracic duct to study the change in the lymph during diseases.

3.3 Rats do not have a gallbladder, so we may collect bile from their bile ducts directly in studying bile functions during the diseases.

3.4 Rats have well-developed pituitary-adrenal system, therefore they are often utilised in studying stress response and endocrine functions. They also have high-level neural activities, so rats are widely used in neurosis researches.

3.5 Rats are sensitive to inflammation, hence we often observe the anti-inflammatory effects of certain drugs on rat ankle arthritis models.

3.6 Rat models are also often used in long-term toxicity experiments of new drugs.

4. Guinea Pigs

Guinea Pigs are particularly sensitive to histamine, therefore they are the most ideal lab animal for screening antiasthmatic drugs and antihistamines. Guinea pigs are also susceptible to mycobacterium tuberculosis, therefore we can screen anti-tuberculosis drugs with them. Their heart and ileum are also common experimental specimens.

5. Rabbits

There are three main breeds of lab rabbits in China as listed below:

The Chinese rabbit with pure white fur and red eyes, is a long-term breed in China. Adult Chinese rabbits weigh from 1.5 to 3.5 kg.

Cyan purple blue rabbits are silver-grey. Adult rabbit weighs from 2.5 to 3.5 kg.

Big-ear white rabbits (Japanese big-ear white) have pure white fur, red eyes, large ears, clear blood vessels, and are convenient for intravenous injection and blood sampling. Adult big-ear white rabbits weigh from 4 to 6 kg.

We can replicate many pathological models on rabbits, such as edema, inflammation, electrolyte disorders, acid-base balance disorders, etc.

Compared with other lab animals, rabbit models have these features below:

5.1 Rabbits are low-cost, docile, easy to raise and reproduce, and it's not difficult to find similar rabbits for the control group. Hence, we mainly choose rabbits when the experiment requires relative large animals.

5.2 In terms of blood circulation, although rabbits' blood vessels are thinner than that of dogs, we can still easily trace their blood pressure, including carotid artery pressure and femoral artery pressure, etc. However, their vascular function is not as good as that of cats and dogs, so they are not the ideal model for observing blood pressure responses. Besides, reflex failure and unstable blood pressure response may occur on rabbits, hence you should be gentle while performing surgery on them.

As the decompression nerve of dog lies in the mixed nerves (vagus sympathetic trunk) in the neck, that nerve of rabbit lies independently, which is very convenient for us to observe its effect on heart and vascular system. Meanwhile, isolated rabbit's heart can still beat for a while. Therefore, it's suitable to observe the effect of harmful factors on mammalian hearts with them. Isolated rabbit ears can also be used as a model to observe the effect of harmful factors on blood vessels.

5.3 Rabbits are also suitable for studying fever, antipyretic drugs and determining heat sources.

5.4 Digestive system: as rabbits are herbivore and their digestive system is different than that of human, especially they don't have vomiting reflex, rabbits cannot be used in studying digestive drugs.

5.5 Adult female rabbits are easy to induce ovulation under stimulations, so we may choose them to study contraceptives.

5.6 Rabbits have similar skin reactions with human to irritants, so they are suitable for observing local skin effects of drugs.

5.7 Others: rabbits are not sensitive to histamines, and histamine injection can not drop their blood pressure but may boost it. Hence, we should not replicate the an aphylactic shock model on rabbits by histamine injections.

6. Cats

Cats have similar head shapes to rabbits, but brain of cats is around 2 times larger than that of rabbit's, hence cat models are suitable for observing the effect of drugs that require intracerebral administrations. Cats also have a more stable blood pressure response, so they are suitable for observing the effect of drugs on blood pressure.

7. Dogs

Dogs can also be used to replicate many pathological models, such as edema, inflammation, electrolyte disturbances, acid-base balance disorders, hypoxia, etc.

Compared with other lab animals, dog models have these features below:

7.1 Dogs have great compliance and we may perform operations in their awake state if necessary. Therefore, they are suitable for chronic experiments, such as hypertension, radiation sickness and neurosis.

7.2 Dogs have large body and strong tolerance to operations, so they are ideal models for surgeries that are not suitable for small animals, such as gastric fistula, Pavlov pouch, intestinal fistula, bladder fistula, etc., in order to observe the change in metabolism functions of specific organs.

7.3 Dogs have developed blood circulation system and thick blood vessels, and can withstand traumas to a certain level. Therefore, dog models are often applied in directly tracing systemic arterial blood pressure, pulmonary arterial pressure, etc., in order to observe the the change of blood pressure under shock, DIC, acute heart failure and so on. Beside, as dogs have large hearts, it is easier to ligate the coronary artery and replicate myocardial infarction models on them.

7.4 Dogs have developed nerve system and similar digestive process to human, so they are often applied in observing the change of nerve and digestive systems under some diseases.

7.5 Dogs have very sensitive vomiting reflex, so they are often used in observing the vomiting and antiemetic effect of drugs.

7.6 Preclinical toxicity studies of new drugs, etc. The reasons for dogs as the first choice of non-rodent animals for pre-clinical chronie toxicity tests of new drugs are as following: firstly, they are so easy to domesticate to cooperate well in long-term experiments; secondly, their biological transformation of subjects is close to that of humans; moreover, they are commonly used to be experimental animals, so there are a large number of historical data as reference.

8. Monkeys

Monkeys are advanced animals, similar to human. They have well-developed nerve system, hence we can observe the effect of drugs on behaviour on them. Monkeys also have a menstrual cycle that is same with human, so they are the first choice in studying reproduction. In addition, preclinical toxicity evaluations of new drugs also require monkey models.

第一章　实验动物基本知识

知识要求

1. 掌握药理实验选用动物的基本要求及常用实验动物的特点。

2. 熟悉实验动物的种类及用途。

能力要求

学会根据实验目的正确选用实验动物。

一、实验动物的要求

药理学实验研究通常采用动物进行实验，根据不同的实验目的选用相应合格的实验动物，对实验研究的可靠性和准确性非常重要。

实验动物按照微生物学控制标准分为4个等级：①普通动物（conventional animals，CV）是在微生物学控制上要求最低的动物，要求不携带人畜共患病和动物烈性传染病的病原。②清洁动物（clean animals，CL）除了普通动物应排除的病原体外，不能携带对动物危害大和对科学研究干扰大的病原体。③无特定病原体动物（specific pathogen free animals，SPF）简称SPF动物，是指动物体内无特定的微生物和寄生虫存在，比清洁动物需控制或排除的微生物和寄生虫的种类更多。④无菌动物（germ free animals，GF）和悉生动物（gnotobiotic animals，GN）无菌动物是指用现有的检测技术在动物体内外的任何部位均检不出任何微生物和寄生虫的动物。悉生动物又叫知菌动物或已知菌丛动物，是指在无菌动物体内植入一种或几种已知微生物的动物。药理实验可选用普通动物，科学研究必须用清洁级以上的实验动物。

实验中选用动物，除根据各种实验动物的特点以及复制动物疾病模型的经验，还应逐一考虑下述问题：所要求的疾病模型能否复制成功及成功率大小；采用的方法和所观察指标是否简单易行；实验结果稳定一致的程度；动物是否便于管理；所获得的结果和人的临床情况相似性的大小；须耗费的人力、物力、财力等。只有对这些因素进行综合考虑，比较以后，才能确定采用何种动物较为合适。在教学上，不但要考虑以上这些问题，还应考虑教学效果，才能满足实验的目的和要求。

二、实验动物的选择

药理实验常用的哺乳动物种类有：小鼠、大鼠、豚鼠、兔、狗、猫、猴。它们的生理特性和人接近。常用的实验动物简介如下：

1.青蛙和蟾蜍 易饲养，其心脏在离体情况下仍能较持久地节律搏动，常用于心功能不全、致病因素对心脏的直接作用等模型。其坐骨神经腓肠肌标本可用来观察药物对周围神经、横纹肌或神经肌肉接头的作用，并用于局麻药和肌松药的研究。蛙舌和肠系膜是观察炎症和微循环变化的良好标本。另外，蛙类也可用于水肿和肾功能不全的实验。

2. 小鼠 易大量繁殖，适用于需要大量动物的实验，如药物半数致死量测定和药物的初筛实验。小鼠妊娠期仅20天，繁殖能力很强。

小鼠能用于复制许多病理过程和疾病，如水肿、炎症、缺氧、多种恶性肿瘤、肉瘤、白血病、多种传染病、慢性气管炎、心室纤颤、寄生虫感染疾病等。也常用于研究避孕药和抗肿瘤药物的筛选与药物致癌性的研究。

小鼠复制疾病模型，较于其他实验动物具有以下主要特点：

（1）小鼠价格低廉，便于大量繁殖，对动物实验同种、纯种、性别和年龄的要求比较容易满足，生活条件也容易控制，是实验室最常用的一种动物。因而只要符合实验要求，应尽量采用。其次，小鼠适合于需要大量动物的实验，容易满足统计学的要求。例如胰岛素、促肾上腺皮质激素的生物效价的测定，毒物半数致死量的测定等。

（2）小鼠对许多疾病有易感性，因而适用于研究这类疾病。例如血吸虫病、疟疾、流感、脑炎等。小鼠的纯种品系甚多，每品系有其独特的生物特性，对某些疾病易感。例如C3HA系对癌瘤敏感，C57系则抗癌。因此，纯系小鼠广泛应用于各种肿瘤的研究。

（3）小鼠因为器官较小，当研究指标主要为组织学观察特别是电镜观察时，可节约人力、物力。例如用小鼠研究慢性气管炎时肺的变化。

（4）小鼠具有发达的神经系统，能应用于复制神经官能症模型。

（5）小鼠对外界环境适应性差，不耐冷热，比较娇嫩，因此，做实验时要耐心细致，动作要轻，不然会干扰实验结果。

3. 大鼠　除形体比小鼠大外，其他方面与小鼠相似。大鼠能用于复制许多病理过程，如水肿、炎症、缺氧、休克、弥漫性血管内凝血（DIC）、胆固醇肉芽肿、心肌梗死、肝炎、肾性高血压、各种肿瘤等。用大鼠复制疾病模型较其他实验动物有以下主要特点：

（1）大鼠和小鼠相似，易于大量繁殖，对动物实验同种、纯种、性别和年龄的要求，比较容易满足，生活条件也容易控制，适用于需求量大且小鼠不满足实验要求的实验，如不对称亚硝胺口服或胃肠道外给药，能诱发大鼠食道癌，而小鼠则很少引起食道癌，因而，在这种情况下，采用大鼠作为实验模型较为合适。

（2）大鼠体型较小鼠大，对须用较大体型的动物实验，选用大鼠较为适合。例如，大鼠可用于直接记录血压，其血压反应比家兔好。大鼠可用于研究休克、DIC时血液循环变化实验。大鼠后肢可用于肢体血管灌流实验，其心脏可用于离体心脏实验。从大鼠胸导管采集淋巴液能研究疾病时淋巴液的变化。

（3）大鼠无胆囊，因此，常用大鼠胆管收集胆汁，用于疾病时胆汁功能的研究。

（4）大鼠的垂体–肾上腺系统功能很发达，常用于应激反应和肾上腺、垂体等内分泌功能实验；大鼠的高级神经活动发达，因此，也广泛用于神经官能症的研究。

（5）大鼠对炎症反应比较灵敏，常作为踝关节炎模型观察药物的抗炎作用。

（6）大鼠还常用于新药长期毒性实验。

4. 豚鼠　对组胺特别敏感，是筛选平喘药和抗组胺药最理想的实验动物。豚鼠还易被结核杆菌感染，常用于抗结核病药的筛选。其离体心脏和回肠也是常用的实验标本。

5. 家兔　家兔品种很多，目前我国实验用的家兔主要有以下三种：①中国白兔，毛色多为纯白，红眼睛，是我国长期培育的一种品种，成年兔体重1.5~3.5 kg。②青紫兰兔（又称山羊青兔或金基拉兔），毛色银灰色，成年兔体重2.5~3.5 kg。③大耳白兔（又称日本大耳白），毛色纯白，红眼睛，两耳长大，血管清晰，便于静脉注射和采血，成年兔体重4~6 kg。

家兔能用于复制许多病理过程和疾病，如水肿、炎症、电解质紊乱、酸碱平衡紊乱、失血、出血性休克、DIC、肺癌、动脉粥样硬化、高脂血症、心律失常、慢性肺心病、慢性肺动脉高压、肺水肿、肝炎、胆管炎、阻塞性黄疸、肾性高血压、肾小球性肾炎、急性肾功能衰竭等。

家兔复制的疾病模型较其他常用实验动物有以下主要特点：

（1）价格较低，性情温顺、易饲养，繁殖率高，容易选到条件类似的对照组兔。因此，当实验中必须用较大体型动物时，常用家兔。

（2）在血液循环方面，家兔血管虽较狗的血管略细，但很容易直接描记颈动脉压、股动脉压、肺小动脉楔压、中心静脉压等。兔的血管系统功能较猫、狗差，用来观察血压反应不如狗、猫。手术时，兔易发生反射性衰竭，血压反应不稳定，故给兔做手术时，动作要轻。狗的减压神经在颈部，存在于混合神经(迷走交感神经干)中，而兔的减压神经是独立走向的，便于观察减压神经对心血管系统的作用。家兔心脏在离体情况下，搏动很久，是观察有害因子对哺乳类动物心脏直接作用较合适的一种模型。离体兔耳，又可作为观察有害因子对血管直接作用的一种模型。

（3）家兔适宜于研究发热、解热药和检查致热源的实验。

（4）家兔是草食动物，消化系统与人类相差较远，缺乏呕吐反射，所以不能用家兔作消化系统方面的研究。

（5）成年雌兔易诱发排卵，常用于避孕药的研究。

（6）家兔皮肤对刺激物的反应接近于人，适应于观察药物对皮肤的局部作用。

（7）其他：家兔对组胺不敏感，注射组胺后并不产生血压下降反应，甚至出现升压反应，因此，对家兔注射大量组胺，并不能构建过敏性休克模型。

6. **猫**　猫和兔的头型比较一致，头部表面与脑的部位有固定的对应关系，但猫脑比兔脑大一倍，更适用于脑内给药观察药物的作用。猫的血压反应比兔稳定，更适合观察药物对血压的影响。

7. **狗**　狗能用于复制许多病理过程和疾病，如水肿、炎症、电解质紊乱、酸碱平衡障碍、缺氧、休克、DIC、心律失常、肺动脉高压，肝淤血、实验性腹水和肾性高血压等。

用狗复制疾病模型较其他常用实验动物有下述主要特点：

（1）易于驯养，经训练后能很好配合，可使狗在清醒状态下进行实验，因而适用于慢性实验，如高血压、放射病和神经官能症等。

（2）对手术的耐受性较强，体型大，常用于许多小型实验动物不适宜的手术，例如，胃瘘、巴浦洛夫小胃、肠瘘、膀胱瘘、胆囊瘘和颈动脉桥等。待动物从这些手术创伤中恢复，再复制胃炎、肾炎、肠炎、肝炎或高血压等疾病，以观察相应器官的功能代谢变化。

（3）血液循环比较发达、血管口径粗、耐受一定创伤，常用于直接描记体循环动脉血压、肺循环动脉压、肺小动脉楔压、中心静脉压、门静脉压和各内脏静脉压等，以观察休克、DIC、急性心力衰竭、窒息、失血、急性死亡和复苏情况下的压力变化；又由于狗心脏较大，手术结扎冠状动脉较容易，故常用来复制心肌梗死模型。

（4）狗具有发达的神经系统和与人相似的消化过程，常用于观察疾病时神经系统和消化系统的功能变化。

（5）狗呕吐反应很灵敏，常用于观察药物的致吐和镇吐作用。

（6）新药临床前毒性实验等。狗易于训养，在长期试验过程中能较好地配合，其对受试物的生物转化与人体接近，而且作为常用的实验动物，有大量历史对照数据，因此，作为新药临床前长期毒性试验的非啮齿类首选动物。

8. 猴　是接近于人类的高级动物。神经系统比较发达，常用于观察药物对行为的影响。猕猴的月经周期和人一样，是研究生殖课题的首选动物。另外，新药临床前毒性评价，也需要用猴作为实验动物。

Section 2   Basic Skills in Animal Experiments

~ ~ · ~ · ~ · ~ · ~ · ~ · ~ · ~ · ~ · ~ · ~ · ~ · ~ · ~ · ~ · ~ · ~ · ~ ·

Knowledge

1. Operation skills in animal experiments.
2. The anatomy structure of mice.

Skill

1.Gender identification, numbering, capture, drug administration, blood sampling and execution of common lab animals, mainly including rats, mice and rabbits.

2. Rationally use surgical instruments.

~ ~ · ~ · ~ · ~ · ~ · ~ · ~ · ~ · ~ · ~ · ~ · ~ · ~ · ~ · ~ · ~ · ~ · ~ ·

Methods of Gender Identification, Numbering and Dehairing Lab Animals

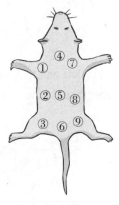

Figure 1.2.1   Marks for Mice Numbering

1. Gender Identification

Mice and Rats: you can mainly identity the gender by the distance between the genital and anus. The urethral orifice of male mouse or rat is relatively far from the anus, and you may see a scrotum, even testicles inside especially in hot environments. However, the vagina of female mouse or rat is closer to the anus, and it has no scrotum. You may also find nipples on their belly.

Guinea pigs: similar with mice and rats.

Rabbits: you can find the scrotum with a testicle on each side near the cloacae of male rabbits, even the penis when you press their genital area with your fingers. As for the female rabbit, you may find 5 pairs of nipples in their abdomen.

The gender of other animals are mainly easy to identify.

2. Numbering Lab Animals

You may hang a number plate on the ear or neck of large animals, such as monkeys, dogs, cats, etc.

We mainly use the dyeing method to number mice, rats and rabbits. Generally, apply 1% picric acid solution (yellow) or 55% neutral red solution (red) to different parts of the animal to represent different numbers. The numbering principle is to start marking from left to right, and front to tail (Fig. 1.2.1). If there are more than 10 animals in a group, you may use 2 numbering colours, one of which represents the single digit and the other one represents the tens digit. You can also mark them on different parts with the same colour, as long as you can identify them.If necessary, you may punch a hole on different parts of the rabbit's ear to number them.

3. Dehairing Animals

Cutting: fix the animal, then cut off the fur on the administration or surgical site. Do not pinch the fur, or you may hurt the animal. The removed fur should be discarded in a large beaker with water inside.

Chemical shaving: we commonly use 8% sodium sulphide solution as the fur remove agent in pharmacology experiments. You may cut the animal's fur on the surgical site a bit shorter, then apply a thin layer of this agent with a cotton ball. Afterwards, wash the surgical site with warm water 2 to 3 minutes later, then dry it with gauze.

Holding Lab Animals

1. Frogs and Toads

You can hold a frog or a toad with your left hand, clamp its left foreleg with your index and middle fingers. Straighten its lower limbs, then fix them between your left ring and little fingers with your right hand (Fig. 1.2.2).

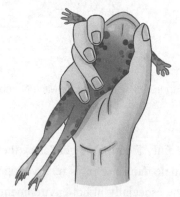

Figure 1.2.2   Catch and Hold a Toad

When destroying the brain or spinal cord of a frog or a toad, hold its head with your left index and middle fingers, then pierce the probe into their cranial cavity through the foramen magnum. Afterwards, swing the probe to destroy its brain. If necessary, pierce the probe into its spinal canal to destroy the spinal cord.

You can also follow your own handedness.

2. Mice

Double hand method: pick up the mouse's tail with your right hand, then place the mouse on a squirrel cage (or an other rough surface), and gently pull its tail. Next, the mouse will fix itself on the surface.Afterwards, quickly pinch its skin around the head and neck with your thumb and index fingers, then fix its tail on the ulnar side of your palm with your little and ring fingers (Fig. 1.2.3).

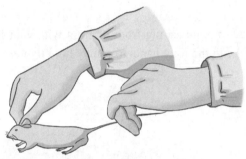

Figure 1.2.3   Catch and Hold a Mouse with Two Hands

One hand method: grasp the mouse's tail with your left thumb and index fingers, then clamp the base of its tail with your palm and little finger. Afterwards, pinch its skin around the head and neck with your left thumb and index finger (Fig. 1.2.4).

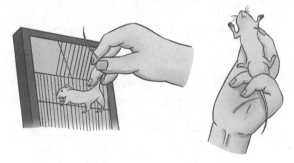

Figure 1.2.4   Catch and Hold a Mouse with One Hands

3. Rats

Rats are similar to mice, but they are easily irritated and may bite you sometimes. Hence, wear a protective glove when catch and hold a rat. Grasp the rat's tail with your right hand, then hold its head with left thumb and index finger. Afterwards, hold its spine and abdomen with your palm and other fingers. Do not pinch its neck, or you may strangle the rat (Fig. 1.2.5).

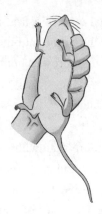

Figure 1.2.5   Catch and Hold a Rat

4. Guinea Pigs

Holds the upper body of a guinea pig from its front with your left hand, and grasp its hind limbs or support its butt with the right hand. You may hold light guinea pigs with just one hand as well (Fig. 1.2.6).

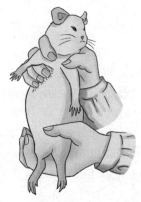

Figure 1.2.6   Catch and Hold a Guinea Pig

5. Rabbits

Grasp the rabbit's skin of its neck, and gently lift it. Support the butt or abdomen of the rabbit with the other hand, making it sit or lie on your arm. You must not lift its ears (Fig. 1.2.7).

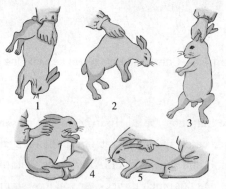

Figure 1.2.7   Catch and Hold a Rabbit

1, 2 and 3 are all wrong, whereas 4 and 5 are correct.

6. Cats

Gently call and caress the cat, then grab its skin on the neck with one hand and that on its back with the other hand. For bad-tempered cats, you may need cloth bag, net and gloves.

7. Dogs

You may put a muzzle on docile dogs, then fasten it with a rope on the neck behind its ears. For bad-tempered dogs, you may clamp the dog's neck with a long handle, then put a muzzle on it. You should also fasten the muzzle with a rope, tying around the lower jaw and the back of its neck (Fig. 1.2.8).

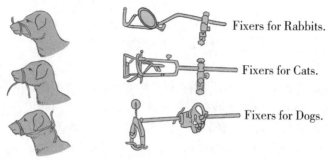

Fixers for Rabbits.

Fixers for Cats.

Fixers for Dogs.

Figure 1.2.8   Steps of Fixing a Dog's Mouth & Animal Head Fixers for Rabbits, Cats and Dogs

In acute experiments, put the anaesthetized dog in its supine position, and fix its limbs on the operating table. Afterwards, remove the muzzle and rope, and put a metal stick through its mouth on the tongue. Then, pull its tongue outside to prevent suffocation. Finally, tie the dog's mouth with a rope around the stick, and fix it on the operating table.

Dosing Lab Animals

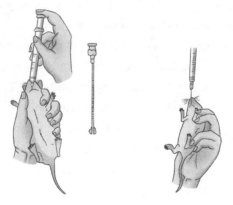

Figure 1.2.9   Dosing a Mouse or a Rat by Gavage

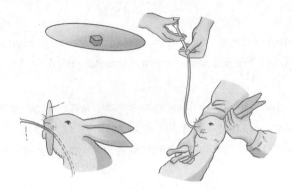

Figure 1.2.10   Dosing a Rabbit by Gavage

1. Gavage

Mice: hold the mouse with your left hand, keeping its head up and neck straight, and its belly facing you. Do not hold it too tight or it may suffocate. Insert the gavage needle into its mouth through the corner of it with your right hand, keeping the tube aligned with the esophagus. Afterwards, gently insert the needle into its esophagus for 2 to 3 centimetres along the palate (Fig. 1.2.9). Immediately remove the gavage needle and try again later when feel abnormal resistance through the syringe, to avoid breaking the mouse's esophagus or trachea, which can be lethal. If the mouse breathes normally and looks calm after the insertion, especially its lips are not cyanotic, you can inject the drug into its stomach.

Rats: similar with mice. If necessary, an assistant can fix the rat's hind limbs and tail. The gavage needle for rat is about 6 to 8 cm long and 1.2 mm in diameter, with a smooth or spherical tip. To avoid inserting the needle into its trachea, you may withdraw the syringe first when you have put the needle inside, if there's no air withdrawn, you can inject the drug into its stomach.

Rabbits: dosing a rabbit by gavage requires a teamwork of at least two people. One person fix the rabbit's body, grasp its forelimbs, and keep its head slightly tilted back. The other person place a gag in the rabbit's mouth, then gently rotate the gag and fix its tongue under it. Afterwards, insert a #8 urinary catheter into the rabbit's esophagus through the hole in the gag, along the upper palate of the rabbit for 15 to 18 cm. The intubation should be smooth, and the rabbit should breath normally and not struggle during the gavage, indicating the catheter is inserted into the stomach. Otherwise, you must remove the tube and try again. In order to make sure the tube is not in the trachea, put the end of it into a cup of water, then you can inject the drug only when no bubble escapes from the tube. After the administration, inject some air into the tube to push the remaining drugs in the tube into the rabbit's stomach(Fig. 1.2.10). Afterwards, slowly pull out the tube and remove the gag.

You may also use a rabbit case to fix the rabbit.

Guinea pigs: the process is similar with mice and rats when using a gavage needle, or similar with rabbit when using a urinary catheter.

Cats and dogs: the process is similar with rabbits, but using larger tools. Be careful of scratching or biting during the gavage.

2. Subcutaneous Injection

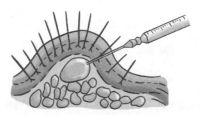

Figure 1.2.11 Dosing a Mouse by Subcutaneous Injection Epidermis/ Dermis/ Subcutaneous Tissue

Mice: dosing mice by subcutaneous injection may require the teamwork of two people. One person fixes the mouse by holding its tail and the skin on its head. The other person lifts the skin on its back with a hand, then pierces the syringe into the mouse's skin with the other hand. If the syringe is easy to swing, indicating that the needle is indeed under the skin, then inject the drug (Fig. 1.2.11).When pulling out the needle, pinch the injection site for a while to avoid leakage.

You may also do that on your own. Place the mouse on a rough surface and hold its tail with a hand. While the mouse is crawling forward, pinch the skin on its neck, forming a triangular socket, then quickly pierce the needle into this site with the other hand and inject the drug.

Rats: similar with mice, but inject on their back or outer thigh.

Guinea Pigs: usually inject under at inner thigh. One person fixes the guinea pig on the table, the other person fixes its hind limbs and pierces its skin with a syringe. After confirming the needle is indeed under the skin, inject drugs. Afterwards, gently press the injection site for a while to prevent leakage.

Rabbit: usually inject under their back neck skin. Lift the skin of the rabbit's back neck and make it wrinkle into a triangle, then pierce the skin and inject drugs into that site.

Cats: inject on their buttock.

Dogs: inject on their back neck.

3. Intramuscular Injection

Mice and Rats: as they have fewer muscles, we seldom dosing them by intramuscular injections. If necessary, similar with the subcutaneous injection, one person fixes the mouse, the other person fixes its hind limbs then injects the drug into its lateral thigh muscle.

Guinea Pigs, Rabbits, Cats and Dogs: injection into their buttock or thigh muscles.

4. Intraperitoneal Injection

Mice: fix the mouse and keep its belly upside, then pierce the skin of it at its lower left or right abdomen towards its head with the needle at a 45° angle to the skin. Do not hurt it's bladder in this process. After puncturing into the abdominal cavity, when you may feel it is 'empty' inside, inject the drug. Do not insert the needle at some sites too high or into some organs to avoid hurting the mouse.

Other Lab Animals: similar with mice.

5. Intravenous Injection

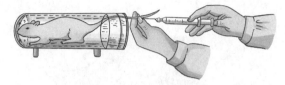

Figure 1.2.12   Dosing a Mouse by Intravenous Injection

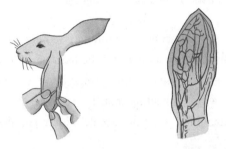

Figure 1.2.13   Dosing a Rabbit by Injecting into the Ears Vein

Mice: mainly inject into their tail vein. Fix the mouse in a special tube and keep its tail outside (Fig. 1.2.12). Make the tail fully congested by soaking it in 75% ethanol or 45℃ warm water for 30 seconds.

Hold its tail with your thumb and index finger, then insert needle into a vein on one side of the tail, keeping it almost parallel to the vein, and inject the drug. If the needle is indeed in the vein, the injection site will not turn white and you won't feel much resistance during the injection, otherwise you should pull out the needle and try again on the other vein. If possible, inject at distal sides of the tail in case of failure, and they are relatively easier to inject. Afterwards, press the injection site to stop bleeding.

Rats: similar with mice. You may also anesthetize the rat first and incise its skin to inject into the femoral or sublingual vein.

Rabbits: mainly inject into their auricular vein.

Dehair the injection site and sterilise it with an alcohol cotton ball, then pinch the tip of the rabbit's ear and place your index finger under it. Afterwards, pierce the needle into the auricular vein from the distal side and inject the drug (Fig. 1.2.13).

If the needle is indeed in the vein, the injection site won't turn swelling and you won't feel much resistance during the injection, otherwise you should pull out the needle and try again on the other side. Afterwards, press the injection site to stop bleeding.

Guinea Pig: inject into their lateral foot vain.

One person holds the guinea pig and fixes its hind leg. The other person dehairs the injection site and sterilises it with an alcohol cotton ball, making the vein obvious, then pierces a intravenous infusion needle for paediatric use that attached to a syringe into the vein. Inject the drug if after finding blood flowing back in the needle. Afterwards, press the injection site to stop bleeding. If necessary, expose their external jugular vein or femoral vein for injection after anesthetization.

Cat: put the cat into a fixing bag or cage, and take out one of its forelimbs, then tighten the upper elbow joint with a rubber band to congest the subcutaneous vein. Next, Dehair and sterilise the injection site, then insert the needle into the blood vessel from the end of the forelimb. After confirming it's in the vein, loosen the rubber band and inject the drug. You may also dosing the cat via the femoral hind limb vein after anesthetization.

Dogs: inject into their small saphenous vein in hind limbs without anesthesia. Dehair and sterilise the injection site, then tighten the upper elbow joint with a rubber band to congest the subcutaneous vein (Fig. 1.2.14). Afterwards, proximally insert the syringe, and inject the drug after finding blood flowing back in the needle.

You may also dose the dog by injecting into the forelimb subcutaneous cephalic vein, which is on the dorsal side of forelimbs. Dehair and sterilise the injection site, tighten the upper elbow joint to congest the vein (Fig. 1.2.15). Afterwards, inject drug into the blood vessel when the needle is indeed in the vein.

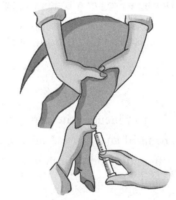

Figure 1.2.14　Dosing a Dog by Injecting into the Small Saphenous Vein

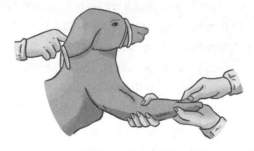

Figure 1.2.15　Dosing a Dog by Injecting into the Forelimb Subcutaneous Cephalic Vein

6. Lymphatic Sac Injection

There are many lymph sacs under the skin of frogs and toads, such as submandibular sac, breast sac, femoral sac, etc. (Fig. 1.2.16), which absorb drugs well. As the skin of frogs and toads is inelastic, drugs may leak via the pinhole. Therefore, you should not inject drug into the lymphatic sac through the skin, but through the muscle layer. For example, when performing chest sac injection, you may pierce the needle through the bottom of the frog's mouth. As for the femoral sac injection, you can pierce the needle into its calf, reaching the thigh via the knee joint to avoid leakage.

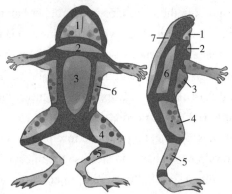

Figure 1.2.16   Dosing a Frog or a Toad by Lymphatic Sac Injection

1. Submandibular lymph sac   2. Chest lymph sac   3. Abdominal lymph sac   4. Femoral lymph sac   5. Tibial lymph sac
6. Side lymph sac   7. Back lymph sac

Blood Collection

The quality of blood sampling influences the experiment result, as we usually collect animal blood samples for biochemical analysis and other purposes in pharmacology studies. Meanwhile, we should apply different blood collection methods on different animals and for different purposes.

1. Mice and Rats

Tail: fix the mouse in a special tube and keep its tail outside. Cut off the tip of it (for 1 to 2 mm for mice, and 5 to 10 mm for rats), then press the tail from the base of it with your thumb and index finger, then collect blood from the wound. You may collect 0.1 ml and 0.5 ml of blood from mice and rats each time, respectively. To collect blood again, just cut off the blood scab. This method is suitable for multiple-time blood collections.

Note: you should only cut of the tip of their tails, or there will be less bleeding.

Eye Socket: fix the mouse, keep its head down and and protrude its eyeball. Clamp the root of the eyeball with a curved forceps, then rapidly remove the eyeball. Afterwards, blood will gush out from the wound for about 4% to 5% of the mouse's body weight. This method is suitable for one-time large amount of blood collection.

Posterior Eye Venous Plexus: fix the mouse and protrude its eyeball, then pierce a special glass straw into its eye posterior venous plexus along the wall of the inner canthus orbit. Gently rotate it, and you'll find blood in the straw. After the collection, pull out the straw and lightly press the would with a dry cotton ball to stop bleeding. This method is suitable for multiple-time small amount of blood collection.

Neck: fix the mouse's head and neck, and tilt it down, then quickly cut off its head with a very sharp scissor. Immediately collect the blood from its neck. You may collect 1 ml and 8 ml of blood from mice and rats, respectively. However, we seldom use this method.

2. Guinea Pigs

Heart: fix the guinea pig and keep its belly upside, then fix its chest with a thumb on one side of the sternum, and the index and middle finger on the other side. Insert a #7 syringe into its chest perpendicularly at where the apex beats most obviously. When feel heart beats through the needle, slightly pierce in and you'll find blood flowing into the syringe. Afterwards, fix the syringe and draw blood with it. You can get 3 to 5 ml of blood each time. The needle must go straight in and out, and you must not 'explore' with syringe in the chest. However, you are not suggested to take blood by this method again in a short time to avoid lethal heart damage to the guinea pig. This method is suitable for taking a large amount of blood.

3. Rabbits

Ear vein: dehair the rabbit's ear edge, then heat it with a bulb or rub it with 75% alcohol to expand the vein. Afterwards, apply paraffin oil on the ear vein, in order to prevent the blood clotting or spreading. Cut the vein with a thick needle or a blade against the blood flow, then collect the blood. Generally, you may get 2 to 3 ml of blood each time. Next, press the wound with a dry cotton ball to stop bleeding.

Central ear artery: fix the rabbit's ear with a hand, then pierce the needle of a syringe into the central ear artery centripetally with the other hand. You'll find blood flowing into the syringe immediately. You can collect 15 ml of blood each time. As this artery spasms easily, you should fully congest it before the sampling, and quickly finish the collection. Press the wound with a dry cotton ball to stop bleeding after the sampling.

Heart: similar with guinea pigs.

4. Dogs

Cephalic vein and small saphenous vein: fix the dog and dehair its sampling sites, then sterilise them with iodine, filling the vein, then draw out the blood. If necessary, you may also collect blood from the dog's heart, jugular vein or femoral artery.

Ear vein: similar with rabbit. This method is suitable for taking a small amount of blood.

Anaesthetization

In short-term or long-term experiments, animals are often anaesthetised, however the anaesthetics can not only inhibit the animal's central nervous system, but also cause changes in other physiological functions. Therefore, it's significant to select a suitable anaesthetic and anesthesia methods to acquire ideal experiment results according to the experiment purpose and lab animals.

1. Inhalation Anesthesia

We commonly employ ether inhalation anesthesia on mice and rats. Put a cotton ball that soaked with 5 to 10 ml of ether at the bottom of a glass container, then place the animal on the mesh partition within the container. Next, seal the container with a lid immediately. 20 to 30 seconds later, and you'll find the animal anaesthetised. You may also place the cotton ball in a small beaker, then put it on the animal's mouth and nose for anaesthetization.

You may also employ inhalation anesthesia with ether on other lab animals, such as dog, cat, rabbit, chicken, etc. It's relatively safe to anaesthetise animals by ether, as it has a huge difference between its anesthesia dosage and its lethal dose. As the animal may quickly recover from this anaesthetization, inhalation anesthesia is only suitable for short operations.

2. Injection Anesthesia

Injection anesthesia is the most common anesthesia method in pharmacology experiments. We often use barbiturates, urethane and chloralose as the anaesthetic. You should select a suitable anesthesia according to the lab animal, study purpose and operation duration.

Barbiturates are ideal anaesthetics in pharmacology studies, such as phenobarbital or sodium pentobarbital is used for long operations, and sodium pentobarbital and thiopental sodium are used for short operations. Urethane has a strong and rapid effect on animals, however, it can also lower the blood pressure and increase the threshold of respiratory centre of rats and cats. Chloralose can inhibit the motor spinal cord centre without affecting the reflex, enhance the adrenaline-induced uterine excitement, and reduce the effect of parasympathetic nerves.

In intravenous anesthesia, you must determine an accurate dosage, then slowly and uniformly inject the drug. When carry out experiments in winters, the drug should be warmed to the animal's body temperature. After the injection, closely observe the animal's reflex of eyelids, cornea and toe to avoid excessive anesthesia and death. Once find excessive anesthesia, you should take actions as soon as possible to save the animal.

For the application, dosage and preparation of anaesthetics, refer to Appendix 3.

Execution

Frogs and toads: decapitation or destroying their brain and spinal cord with a probe.

Mice and rats: cervical dislocation. Fix the animal's head at a hard surface with your thumb and index finger and grasp its tail with the other hand, then forcefully pull it back to dislocate the spine. Luckily, the animal may die instantly without pain.

Rabbits, cats and dogs: air embolisation. Rapidly inject air into the animal's vein with a large syringe (50 to 100 ml), then it will die from the air embolisation. 10 to 20 ml of air can kill a cat or a rabbit, and 70 to 150 ml may execute a dog.

Lethal anesthesia: inject a lethal amount of anaesthetic, for example, inject 2 to 3 times of the normal dose of pentobarbital sodium to the animal, which can severely inhibit the animal's life centre and cause death.

Mass bloodletting: cut the animal's carotid or femoral artery when it's anaesthetised.

Basic Surgery Skills in Pharmacology Experiments

1. Tissue Incision, Separation and Hemostasis

1.1 Tissue incision

Basic principles for tissue incision in pharmacology experiments are listed below:

1.1.1 Determine the location and size of the surgical incision according to the experiment purpose. For example, cut open an oblique incision on the left back when performing a nephrectomy, and cut open a midline incision on the abdomen when performing a bowel resection surgery.

1.1.2 There are three common knife holding styles for cutting open incisions at different locations (Fig. 1.2.17).

Grip (Fig. 1.2.17A). Hold the knife handle, pinch the notch of it with your thumb and index finger, then focus your strength on the wrist. This style is suitable for cutting a large incision with great force, such as cutting open a long incision on skin or fascia, or cut off a chronic hyperplasia tissues, etc.

Bow-holding style (Fig. 1.2.17B) : the most common knife-holding style.

Press at one-third of the knife's back with your index finger, cutting with strength from the wrist and fingers. This style is suitable for incising skin or peritoneum, and cutting the tissue pinched by forceps.

Pen-holding style(Fig. 1.2.17C): similar to holding a pen.

Focus your strength on the finger, supplemented by the wrist.This style is suitable for small but accurate operations, such as cutting open short incisions, separating blood vessels or nerves, etc.

Precautions

(1) Before the incision, tighten the skin or other tissues around the operation site to make them flat and tight.

(2) The blade should be perpendicular to the tissue. If possible, open the incision by a single cut.

(3) Cut open the tissue layer by layer, and you'd better cut following the skin texture or the tissue fiber.

(4) You should select the incision site at where no important blood vessels or nerve locates, to prevent damaging them.

(5) Choose incision sites that are easy to be covered and fixed or catheterised, in order to avoid the dressing falling off due to the animal's movement.

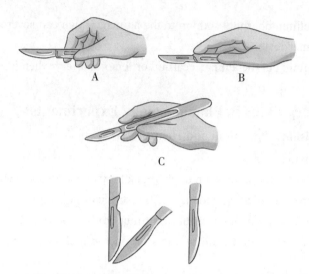

Figure 1.2.17   Knife Holding Styles and Tissue Cutting Method

A. Rip   B. Bow-holding style   C. Pen-holding style

1.2 Tissue separation

Separation aims at fully exposing deep tissues or blood vessels for further operation. Basic principles for separation in pharmacology experiments are listed below:

1.2.1 There are two common separation methods for surgeries at different locations.

1.2.1.1 Sharp separation with knives or scissors: separate tissues by shearing. This method is suitable for separating dense tissues, such as skin, ligaments and fascia, etc.

1.2.1.2 Blunt separation with clamps or handles: separate the tissue by pushing or pulling them away.This method is suitable for loose tissues, such as subcutaneous tissues and muscle-fascial space.

1.2.2 Separate tissues along the tissue gap, which is easier and will cause less bleeding to keep the visual field clear.

Precautions

（1）When separating muscles, you should perform blunt separation in the direction of muscle fibres. When separate it horizontally, clamp at both the upper and lower ends of the incision at first, then ligate these broken ends to prevent bleeding.

（2）Separate nerves or blood vessels following their directions. You must be gentle and careful in this progress to prevent breakage. Avoid excessive horizontal pulling.

1.3 Hemostasis

Bleeding caused by tissue incision or separation must be stopped in time. A fine hemostasis can not only prevent continuous blood loss, but also make the surgical field clear, which is conducive to the operation. Commonly-used hemostasis methods are listed as follow: compression, clamping, ligation, medication and cauterization.

1.3.1 Compression

Compress the bleeding site with dry sterile gauze or cotton balls, mainly to stop capillary bleeding. For bleeding from large blood vessels, you may try compression first, then perform other hemostasis methods.

1.3.2 Clamp

Vertically clamp the end of the bleeding vessel with tip of the hemostat clamp. For small blood vessels, they may stop bleeding after releasing the clamp. As for some large blood vessels, you should clamp them first, then try ligation.

1.3.3 Ligation

A common reliable hemostasis method that can be classified into simple ligation and penetration ligation.

Simple ligation: simply tie the clamped blood vessels or tissues with a thread, which is suitable for compression-ineffective or large blood vessel bleeding. Quickly, firmly and accurately clamp the broken end of the blood vessel with the tip of a hemostat clamp. Afterwards, compress and clean the wound with gauze. When ligating a blood vessel, raise the end of the forceps and wrap the thread under the clamping point first, then keep the clamp flat, and make its tip raised. Slowly loosen the clamp while tying the first knot. Next, tying the second knot when the first one is completely tied (Fig. 1.2.18).

Penetration ligation: pass a thread through the clamped tissue without breaking blood vessels with a surgical needle and then tie the wound. It is suitable for large vessel bleeding and preventing the slippage of ligatures. There are two common penetration methods, including the 8-shaped suture ligation and simple penetration ligation (Fig. 1.2.19).

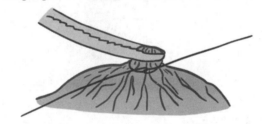

Figure 1.2.18　Simple Ligation Hemostasis

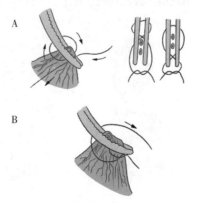

Figure 1.2.19　Penetration Ligation Hemostasis

A. '8' –Shaped Suture Ligation B. Simple Penetration Ligation

1.3.4 Other hemostasis methods

Medication hemostasis: compress the bleeding site with gauze or a cotton ball that soaked with 1% to 2% ephedrine, or 0.005% to 0.01% epinephrine, to constrict the blood vessel and stop bleeding.

Cautery hemostasis: directly burn the broken part of the blood vessel with a electric coagulator or electric knife to coagulate the blood and stop bleeding, which is suitable for small blood vessel bleeding. This method can rapidly stop bleeding and leave no ligatures inside the incision.

2. Suture &Knotting

2.1 Suture

Common suture methods in pharmacology experiments include intermittent suture (as known as nodular suture), mattresssuture, '8'-shaped suture, continuous suture, blanket-edge suture, seromuscular-layer single suture, seromuscular-layer double suture, full-layer inversion suture and purse suture. The suture method is as follows:

2.1.1 Intermittent suture (nodular suture)

Pass the ligature through edges on both sides of the incision, then tie a knot. This method is suitable for skin, subcutaneous tissue, mucous membrane or fascia stitching (Fig. 1.2.20).

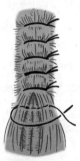

Figure 1.2.20　Intermittent Suture

2.1.2 Mattress suture

Two connected intermittent sutures in opposite directions, which can expose the incision edge, including vertical and parallel style (Fig. 1.2.21).This method is suitable for stitching loose skin or blood vessel.

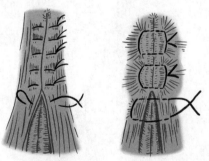

Figure 1.2.21　Mattress Suture (Vertical & Parallel)

2.1.3 '8'-Shaped suture

Two crossed intermittent sutures in opposite directions (Fig. 1.2.22). This method is suitable for stitching fascia or aponeurosis.

2.1.4 Continuous suture

Perform an intermittent suture without cutting the ligature from one end of the incision, and keep doing the same suture until tying the other end of it, then tie a knot. When tying the final knot, you should leave the thread on the other side of the last knot in order to support the last knotting. This method is suitable for stitching inner layer of peritoneum and gastrointestinal anastomosis (Fig. 1.2.23).

2.1.5 Blanket-edge suture (continuous seam suture)

Basically similar to continuous suture, however, you should cross and fix the ligature during the stitching at every knot (Fig. 1.2.24). This method is suitable for stitching inner layers in gastrointestinal surgeries.

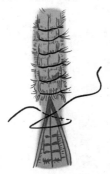 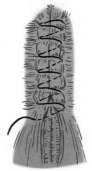

Figure 1.2.22　'8'-Shaped Suture　　Figure 1.2.23　Continuous Suture

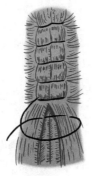

Figure 1.2.24　Blanket-Edge Suture

2.1.6 Seromuscular-layer single suture

Tie knots when the ligature pass through the serosa and the muscular layer on both sides of the incision (Fig. 1.2.25), to pair and fix the serosal membrane together. This method is suitable for stitching outer layers of the gastrointestinal tract.

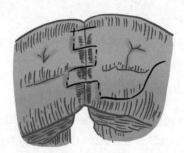

Figure 1.2.25　Seromuscular–Layer Single Suture

2.1.7 Seromuscular-layer continuous suture

Perform a seromuscular-layer single suture at one end of the incision, then continuously suture the seromuscular layer to the other end of it with the same ligature in parallel to the incision (Fig. 1.2.26). This method is suitable for stitching outer layers in gastrointestinal surgeries.

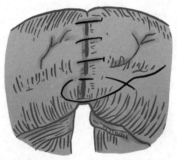

Figure 1.2.26　Seromuscular–Layer Continuous Suture

2.1.8 Full-layer inversion suture

Insert the needle at mucosa and cross the serosa on one side of the incision, knotting in side the cavity and forming an inversion (Fig. 1.2.27). This method is suitable for stitching anterior walls of the gastrointestinal tract.

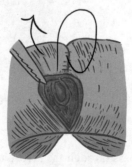

Figure 1.2.27　Full–Layer Inversion Suture

2.1.9 Purse suture

A ringed seromuscular-layer continuous suture (Fig. 1.2.28). This method is suitable for stitching small gastrointestinal wounds to make them inverted.

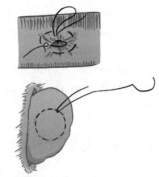

Figure 1.2.28　Purse Suture

Precautions

（1）Completely stop the bleeding and clean all blood clots and free tissues before the suture, flush the would if necessary.

（2）The needle should perpendicularly penetrate or pass through the tissue surface.

（3）Generally, the entrance and exit holes should be beaten least 0.5 to 1.0 cm from the skin incision edge, or 0.2 to 0.5 cm from the incision edge of fascia and other tissues.

（4）Keep needle holes on both sides symmetrical. Do not stitch the wound too tight or too dense, just tightly aligned the incision, to benefit its blood circulation.

（5）Keep anatomical layers respectively aligned when suturing deep incisions.

（6）Knots should be tied at the same side of the incision.

（7）After suturing the skin, align the incision with a forceps. Do not leave the incision edge outside, which may affect recovery.

2.2 Knotting

Correct and firm knotting is a significant part of ligation hemostasis and suture. Skilled knotting may shorten the operation time. Correct knot types in pharmacology experiments include square knot, surgical knot and triple knot, whereas fake knot and slip knot are incorrect and must be avoided (Fig. 1.2.29).

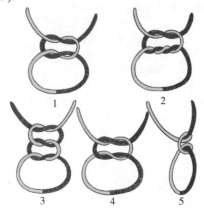

Figure 1.2.29　Knots in Pharmacology Experiments

1. Square knot 2. Surgical knot 3. Triple knot 4. Fake knot 5. Slippery knot

2.2.1 Square knot

Commonly applied in ligation hemostasis and various sutures. Both ends of the thread must be evenly tightened during the ligation to avoid slippery knots.

2.2.2 Surgical knot

Overlap the thread twice when ligating the first line, then knot the second line like ligating a square knot. This kind of knot is relatively firm as it has enlarged friction surface, therefore it's suitable to ligate large blood vessels.

2.2.3 Triple knot

Add another knot on the basis of square knots. This method is suitable for ligating important tissues and large blood vessels.

Commonly used knotting methods are described below:

（1）Single-hand knotting: suitable for various parts, easy and fast (Fig. 1.2.30).

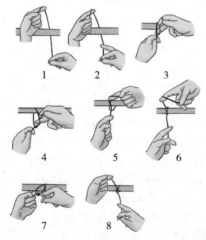

Figure 1.2.30   Single–Hand Knotting

（2）Clamp knotting: suitable for deep tissue sutures, ligation in narrow surgical fields and some delicate operations (Fig. 1.2.31).

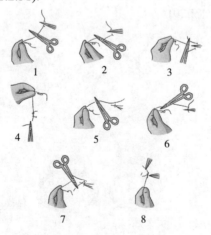

Figure 1.2.31   Clamp Knotting

3. Intravascular Cannula

Multiple blood sampling, drug administration, supplementation of electrolytes and nutrient solutions, etc., always happen in animal experiments, therefore we perform intravascular cannula on them by inserting a nylon or plastic catheter into the animal's blood vessel and connect it to experiment devices.The intravascular cannula is easy to operate and fix, and can maintain for a relatively long period. Most commonly cannulated vessels in experiments are external jugular vein, femoral vein, femoral artery and common carotid artery. All these blood vessels are relatively shallow, large and easy to identify.

3.1 Cannulation into external jugular vein and common carotid artery

Dogs, rabbits and cats have very thick external jugular veins shallowing under their skin on both sides of the neck. However the common carotid artery is located at the outside of their trachea, in front of the sternocleidomastoid muscle, and its ventral surface is covered by the sternohyoid muscle and sternothyroid muscle. The method of cannula into these vessels are described below:

3.1.1 Preparing the operation site

Fix the animal in a supine position on the operating table after anesthetization. Keep its head facing the other side of the cannula. Next, dehair and disinfect the cannula site.

3.1.2 Separating external jugular vein and common carotid artery

Cut open the animal's skin at the midpoint between the sternal notch and the thyroid cartilage. Afterwards, lift up the skin, then you can find the thick dark-purple external jugular vein. You may intubate one of them after the blunt separation (Fig. 1.2.32).

You can also find a even thicker pink pulsing common carotid artery after separating the tissue between the sternohyoid muscle and the sternothyroid muscle, along the sternocleidomastoid muscle. When separating the common carotid artery, you should start at a relatively far place below the thyroid, avoiding cutting the anterior thyroid artery, then gently blunt-separate the connective tissue between the artery and nerves. During the separation, the surgical incision should be moistened with normal saline from time to time, and kept clean. In order to facilitate the arterial cannulation, you should separate the common carotid artery for a certain length. For example, 5 to 6 cm for dogs, 4 to 5 cm for rabbits and cats, and 2 to 3 cm for guinea pigs and rats.

3.1.3 Intubation into external jugular vein and common carotid artery

Firstly, prepare the catheter. Cut a bevel at the insertion end, and connect the other end to an injection needle or infusion device containing anticoagulant solution or saline, then fill the tube with that solution. Afterwards, pass two threads under the separated artery or veins, then ligate the blood vessel at its distal end and gently lift the ligatures to keep the vessel tense. Next, cut a small V-shaped opening on the blood vessel with an ophthalmic scissor. Then, gently insert the prepared catheter through the opening and tightly tie a thread at the proximal end under the insertion port. Afterwards, fix the catheter and put the blood vessel back in place. Try infusing normal saline into the vessel to check if it is unobstructed and whether there is any leakage. When found coagulation, flush it with saline. If there is leakage, ligate the proximal end again. You may suture the incision according to the experiment purpose at this time, leaving the catheter connected to the infusion device.

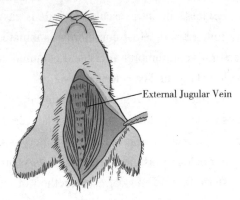

Figure 1.2.32　External Jugular Vein Separation on a Rabbit

Appendix: Anatomical Location and Morphological Characteristics of Main Organs of Mice

1. Lung

The mouse lung includes left and right lobes, of which the right one is divided into four parts (apical lobe, heart lobe, diaphragm lobe and accessory lobe), and the left one has a not-so-deep sulcus on it, which divides it into two sections and looks like a incomplete lobe (Fig. 1.2.33).

2. Heart

The mouse heart is conical, locates near the sternum. Its apex is under the fourth intercostal space. Mice also have large auricles. The mouse's heart and main blood vessels are shown in Fig. 1.2.34.

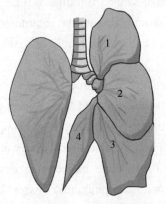
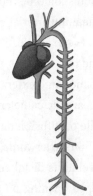

Figure 1.2.33　The Mouse Lung
1. Apical lobe 2. Heart lobe 3. Diaphragm lobe 4. Accessory lobe

Figure 1.2.34　The Mouse Heart and Its Main Blood Vessels

3. Liver

The mouse liver is dark brown and attached to its diaphragm. It is divided into five lobes (lateral left lobe, medial left lobe, lateral right lobe, medial right lobe, and caudate lobe) as it's shown in Fig. 1.2.35.

4. Stomach

The mouse stomach includes cardia, pylorus, stomach fundus and stomach body. The mucosa of its pylorus inner wall is wrinkled as it's shown in Fig. 1.2.36.

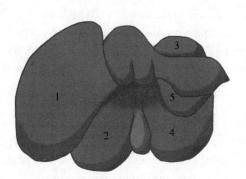

Figure 1.2.35 The Mouse Liver

1. Left lateral lobe 2. Left medial lobe
3. Right lateral lobe 4. Right medial lobe 5. Caudate lobe

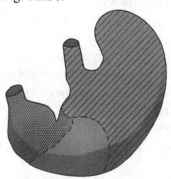

Figure 1.2.36 The Mouse Stomach

5. Intestine

The mouse intestine includes small and large intestines. The small intestine is about 50 to 65 cm long, including duodenum, jejunum and ileum. Whereas the large intestine is about 12 to 17 cm long, including cecum, colon and rectum.

6. Spleen

The mouse spleen lies obliquely on the left side of its stomach. It is dark red, long and flat.

7. Pancreas

The mouse pancreas is pink and locates near the duodenum. The opening of mouse pancreas, common bile duct and duodenum is shown in Fig. 1.3.37.

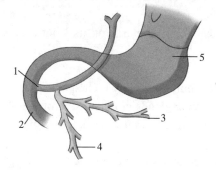

Figure 1.2.37 The Mouse Common bile duct and duodenum

1. Common bile duct 2. Duodenum 3. Anterior pancreatic duct 4. Posterior pancreatic duct 5. Stomach body

8. Kidneys

Mouse's kidneys are a pair of dark-red broad-bean-shaped organs lying on the dorsal wall of the abdominal cavity. The right kidney is slightly higher. There are adrenal glands in front of the kidney, and ureters on the inner side of them connecting to the opening at the back of its bladder.

9. Bladder

The mouse bladder locates at the back of its abdominal cavity and directly leads to the urethra.

10. Testicles

Young male mice has a pair of testicles in their abdominal cavity, which will fall into the scrotum when they got sexually mature. The volume of adult mouse testis is about 8.5mm×5mm×5mm, and its weight is 70 to 90mg. The surface of testicle is a fibrous connective tissue, which contains countless seminiferous tubules to produce sperm.The interstitial tissue of testicles produces androgen.

11. Epididymis

The epididymis consists of many connected thin tubules that temporarily receive and store sperms. The mouse epididymis includes three parts: head, body and tail. The epididymis head is connected to seminiferous tubules. The epididymis body goes down on one side of the testis. Whereas the epididymis tail is connected to the vas deferens. Sperm cell matures while passing through the epididymis. Mature vigorous sperm would be shot into the vagina of a female mouse during mating through the vas deferens that connected to the epididymis.

12. Ovary

Ovary produces eggs. The mouse ovary is a pair of pink mung-bean-shaped organs that locates under each kidney. Adult female mice usually ovulate periodically (for 4 to 5 days) throughout the year except during their pregnancy.

13. Uterus

Female mouse has a bicornuate uterus. Their uterus is a Y-shaped organ including the uterine horn and uterine body. The uterine horn starts at the junction of fallopian tubes and descends along the back of the mouse's body. Two uterine horns meet on at the back of the bladder and forming the uterus.

The uterine body is divided into two parts, the front part is separated by a septum into two separate uterus. The back septum disappears. After the merge of left and right uterus, the cervix gradually forms.The end of their cervix protrudes from the vagina.

14. Vagina

The mouse vagina connects to the uterus on its front part, and the vaginal opening on its back part.

15. The Vas Deferens

The vas deferens is the tubule through which sperm passes. Mouse capillaries merge into urethra under the seminal vesicle glands at dorsal side of the bladder from the epididymis tail. There are countless fertilisable sperms in the vas deferens of an adult male mouse.

16. Fallopian

The fallopian is the tube-structure through which the egg cell is fertilised and passes through. Female mice have two curved fallopian in both sides of their body, locating between the ovary and the uterine horn. Its front opening faces the ovary, and its back end is adjacent to the uterus.

第二章　动物实验基本操作技术

知识要求

1. 掌握动物实验基本操作技术要点。

2. 熟悉小鼠的解剖结构。

能力要求

1. 熟练掌握常用动物（主要是大、小鼠、家兔）性别鉴别、编号、捉拿、给药、取血、处死方法。

2. 掌握手术器械的使用方法。

一、实验动物的性别鉴别、编号及去毛方法

1. 实验动物性别鉴别

小鼠和大鼠：主要通过生殖器与肛门距离远近辨别。雄性尿道口与肛门距离远，可见阴囊，睾丸下垂，热天尤其明显；雌性阴道口与肛门距离较近，无阴囊，成熟雌鼠可见腹部乳头。

豚鼠：方法同大、小鼠。

家兔：雄兔泄殖孔附近可见阴囊，两侧各一睾丸，用拇指、食指按压生殖器部位，雄兔可露出阴茎；雌兔腹部5对乳头明显可见。

其他动物特征明显较易辨别。

2. 实验动物编号

较大动物如猴、狗、猫等可用号码牌固定于耳或颈部。

小鼠、大鼠和兔多采用染色法，一般用1%的苦味酸溶液（黄色）或55%中性红溶液（红色）涂于动物体表不同部位的皮毛处，代表不同号码。标号原则：先左后右，自前到后（图1-2-1）。如10只以上动物做标记，可用两种颜色，一种颜色作为个位数，另一种颜色作为十位数；也可在不同部位标记同一种颜色的组合。方法不尽相同，以能明显区别为原则。如果必须的话，亦可用打孔器在耳朵不同部位做标记。

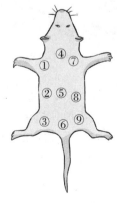

图1-2-1　小鼠标记

3.去毛方法

剪毛法：固定动物，剪刀紧贴动物皮肤，依次将穿刺或手术部位的被毛剪去。注意切勿用手提被毛，否则易剪破皮肤。剪下的被毛放置于盛水的大烧杯中弃去。

化学脱毛法：常用的脱毛剂为8%的硫化钠水溶液。先将动物手术部位的被毛剪短，然后用棉球沾脱毛剂涂一薄层，2~3分钟后用温水洗涤脱毛部位皮肤，再用纱布擦干。

二、实验动物的捉持方法

1.青蛙和蟾蜍 通常用左手握持，以食指和中指夹住左前肢，大拇指压住右前肢，右手将下肢拉直并固定于无名指和小指之间（图1-2-2）。捣毁脑和脊髓时，左手食指和中指夹持青蛙或蟾蜍的头部，右手将探针经枕骨大孔向前刺入颅腔，左右摆动探针捣毁脑组织。如需破坏脊髓，毁脑后退回探针刺入椎管即可。

2.小鼠 双手捉拿法：通常右手提起鼠尾，放在鼠笼（或其他粗糙面）上，向后轻拉其尾，小鼠即固定于鼠笼上，迅速用左手拇指和食指捏住小鼠头颈部皮肤，并以左手小指、无名指压其尾部于手掌尺侧（图1-2-3）。单手捉拿法：只用左手，先用食指和拇指抓住小鼠尾巴后用手掌尺侧和小指夹住尾根部，然后用左手拇指和食指捏住头颈部皮肤（图1-2-4）。

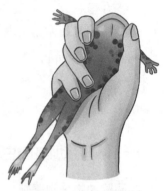

图 1-2-2　蟾蜍的捉拿

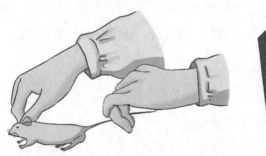

图 1-2-3　小鼠双手捉拿

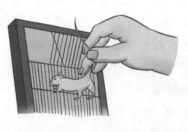

图 1-2-4　小鼠单手捉拿

3. 大鼠 捉持方法与小鼠相似。因大鼠容易被激怒咬人，捉持时左手应戴防护手套。右手抓住鼠尾，再用左手拇指和食指握住头部，其余手指与手掌握住脊部和腹部。注意不要捏其颈部，以防用力过大、过久，造成窒息死亡（图1-2-5）。

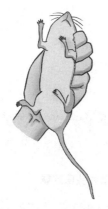 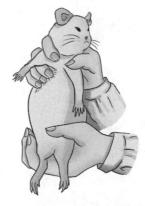

图 1-2-5　大鼠的捉拿　　　　　　　图 1-2-6　豚鼠的捉拿

4.豚鼠　以左手直接从前侧握持前部躯干，右手托住臀部或抓住两后肢。体重小者，可用单手捉持（图1-2-6）。

5.家兔　捉持方法是：一只手抓住兔颈背部皮肤，将兔轻轻提起，另一只手托住臀部或腹部，使兔呈蹲坐姿势或趴于手臂。切不可用手握持双耳提起家兔（图1-2-7）。

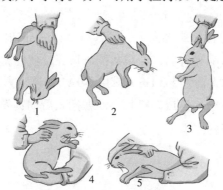

图 1-2-7　家兔的捉拿

1,2,3 均为不正确的捉拿方法；4,5 为正确的捉拿方法

6.猫　捉持方法是轻声呼唤，慢慢将手伸入猫笼，轻抚猫头、颈和背部，一只手抓住颈背部皮肤，另一手抓住腰背部。性情凶暴的猫，要用布袋或网套捉拿，并戴防护手套，以防其利爪和牙齿伤人。

7.狗　对驯服狗，可戴上特制嘴套并用绳带固定于耳后颈部。对凶暴的狗，可用长柄捕狗夹钳住狗的颈部，然后套上嘴套。狗嘴也可用绳带固定，操作时将绳带绕过狗嘴的下颌打结后，再绕到颈后部打结，以防绳带脱落（图1-2-8）。

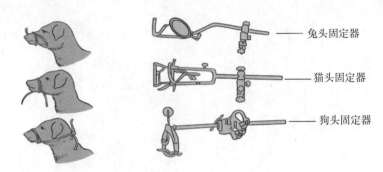

图1-2-8　捆绑狗嘴的步骤及动物头固定器

急性实验时，狗麻醉后呈仰卧位放置，将四肢固定于手术台上，取下嘴套和绳带，将一金属棒经两侧嘴角，穿过口腔压于舌上，将舌拉出口腔，以防窒息。然后再用绳带绕过金属棒绑缚狗嘴并固定于手术台上。

三、实验动物的给药方法

1.灌胃

小鼠：左手捉持小鼠，头部向上，颈部拉直，腹部朝向操作者，但不宜抓得过紧，以免小鼠窒息。右手持灌胃针管，经口角插入口腔，使灌胃针管与食管成一直线，将灌胃针管沿上腭壁缓慢插入食管2~3 cm（图1-2-9）。如遇阻力，立即将灌胃针管抽出另插，以免刺破食道或误入气管，造成动物死亡。如插入后动物安静，呼吸无异常，口唇无发绀现象，即可将药物注入。

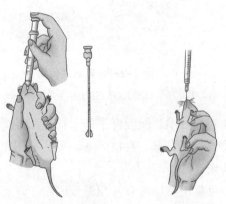

图1-2-9　大鼠、小鼠灌胃

大鼠：左手捉持大鼠，右手持灌胃针管，灌胃方法与小鼠相似。必要时，可有一助手协助固定大鼠的后肢与尾巴。灌胃针管长6~8 cm，直径1.2 mm，尖端平滑或呈球状。为防止插入气管，应回抽注射器针栓，如无空气被抽回，再注入药液。

家兔：给家兔灌胃需二人合作，将家兔躯体固定在兔盒内，左手抓住家兔双耳，固定其头部，右手抓住两前肢，使兔头稍向后仰。另一人将开口器横放于家兔口中，慢慢旋转开口器，将兔舌压住，并固定。将8号导尿管经开口器中央孔，沿家兔上腭壁缓慢插入15~18 cm。插管时感觉顺利，动物不挣扎，也无呼吸困难，表示导尿管插入胃内。为避免导尿管误入气管，可将导尿管的外口端放入清水杯中，无气泡逸出，方可注入药液，再用少量清水冲洗导尿管或注入少量空气，使导尿管内残存药液全部灌入胃中（图1-2-10）。灌胃结束后，慢慢拔出导尿管，取出开口器，也可将家兔置于兔固定盒中按上述步骤进行灌胃。

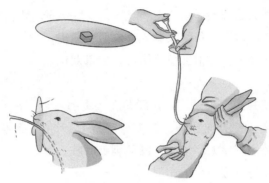

图1-2-10 家兔灌胃

豚鼠：如用灌胃针管，灌胃方法与大鼠相同。如用开口器和导尿管，操作方法与家兔灌胃法相同。

猫和狗：灌胃方法与家兔相同，只是所应用的灌胃器具相应大些。操作时需注意防止动物抓伤或咬伤。

2.皮下注射方法

小鼠：一般需两个人合作。一人左手捏住小鼠头部皮肤，右手拉住小鼠尾巴使小鼠固定。另一人左手提起小鼠背部皮肤，右手持注射器将针头刺入小鼠皮下，稍稍摆动针头，若容易摆动则表明针尖确实位于皮下，注入药液（图1-2-11）。拔针时左手捏住针刺部位片刻，以防药液溢出。

亦可一人操作，将小鼠放在粗糙平面上，左手拉住鼠尾，趁小鼠向前爬动时，捏起颈部皮肤使之呈三角窝状，右手持注射器迅速将针头刺入小鼠皮下，推注药液。

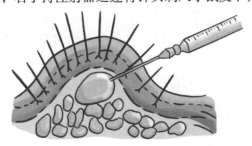

图1-2-11 皮下注射

大鼠：与小鼠皮下注射方法基本相同，注射部位为背部或大腿外侧皮下。

豚鼠：通常在豚鼠大腿内侧皮下注射。操作时一人将豚鼠固定在台上，另一人左手固定注射侧的后肢，右手持注射器刺入皮下，确定针头在皮下后，注射药液。注射完毕后用手指压住刺入部位片刻，以防药液溢出。

家兔：通常选择颈背部皮下注射。操作者左手拇指、食指和中指提起家兔颈背部皮肤，使其皱成三角体，右手持注射器自褶皱下方刺入皮下，松开皮肤注入药液。

猫和狗：猫常注射于臀部皮下，狗可注射于颈部皮下。

3.肌肉注射方法

小鼠和大鼠：两人合作时，一人如同皮下注射方法所述固定动物，另一人左手固定注射侧后肢，右手持注射器，将针头刺入外侧股部肌肉。

豚鼠、家兔、猫和狗：注射部位为臀部和股部肌肉。

4.腹腔注射方法

小鼠：左手捉持并固定小鼠，将腹部朝上，头部下倾，右手持注射器在下腹左侧或右侧（避开膀胱）向头部方向穿刺，针头与皮肤呈45°角，刺入腹腔后（有落空感）注入药液。注意进针部位不要太高太深，以免刺破肝脏。

其他动物腹腔注射方法与小鼠相似。

5.静脉注射方法

小鼠：多采用尾静脉注射。将小鼠固定在特制固定筒内，使鼠尾露在外面（图1-2-12）。用75%乙醇或在45℃左右温水中浸泡30秒，使鼠尾充血。注射时，左手拇指与食指捏持鼠尾，右手持注射器，选择鼠尾两侧静脉，使针头与鼠尾几乎平行，进行静脉穿刺。如推注药液时无阻力，则表明针确在血管内，可持续推完药液；如推注阻力大，局部皮肤发白则表明针头未刺入血管，应重新穿刺。注意静脉穿刺应从鼠尾远端开始，不仅容易穿刺，而且还可以向近端多次穿刺。注射完毕，用手指压住穿刺部位止血。

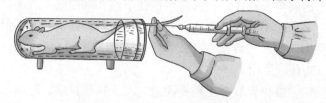

图1-2-12　小鼠尾静脉注射

大鼠：尾静脉注射方法与小鼠相同。亦可将大鼠麻醉，切开皮肤从股静脉穿刺或舌下静脉给药。

家兔：常用耳缘静脉。注射部位去毛并用酒精棉球涂擦，用左手拇指和中指捏住兔耳尖部，以食指垫于耳下，右手持注射器，从静脉远端将针头刺入血管，将药液推入。如推注时有阻力，局部出现肿胀，表明针头不在血管内，应重新注射。注射完毕，用手指压住穿刺部位止血（图1-2-13）。

豚鼠：可选用后脚掌外侧静脉。注射时，一人捉持豚鼠并固定一条后腿，一人剪去注射部位的被毛，用酒精棉球涂擦后脚掌外侧的皮肤，使血管暴露，再将连在注射器上的小儿头皮静脉输液针头刺入血管，有回血即可推注药液。注射完毕后压迫止血。必要时可在麻醉状态下暴露颈外静脉或股静脉注射。

猫：将猫装入固定袋或笼内，取出前肢，用橡皮带扎紧肘关节上部，使前肢皮下头静脉充血，去毛并用酒精消毒，从前肢末端将注射针刺入静脉，确认针头在血管内，即松开橡皮带并注入药液。亦可将猫麻醉后从后肢股静脉给药。

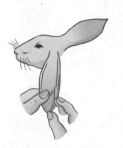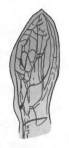

图 1-2-13 家兔耳缘静脉注射

狗：未麻醉的狗可选用后肢小隐静脉。去毛消毒，一人双手紧握注射后肢上部或扎橡皮带（图 1-2-14），使静脉充盈，朝向心端刺入静脉，有回血即可推入药液。

亦可选用前肢皮下头静脉，该血管在前肢脚爪上方背侧的前正位。剪毛消毒后，一人紧捏注射肢体的上端，阻断血液回流，使静脉充盈，一人持注射器作静脉穿刺（图 1-2-15），确认针头在血管内，即可注入药液。

6.淋巴囊注射方法

蛙和蟾蜍：皮下有多个淋巴囊，如颌下囊、胸囊、股囊等（图 1-2-16）。将药液注入囊内吸收良好。由于蛙和蟾蜍皮肤无弹性，药液易从针眼溢出，因此注射时不能通过皮肤直接进入淋巴囊，而应将针头刺入肌层，进入邻近的淋巴囊后再注入药液。如通过胸囊注射时，应将针头刺入口腔，由口腔底部穿过颌下肌层达胸部皮下；通过股囊注射时，应由小腿皮肤刺入，通过膝关节到达大腿部皮下，这样才能避免药液外漏。

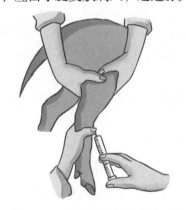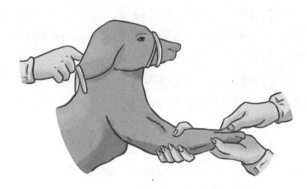

图 1-2-14 狗后肢小隐静脉注射　　　　图 1-2-15 狗前肢皮下头静脉注射

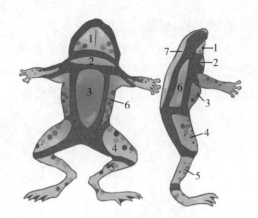

图 1-2-16　蛙及蟾蜍皮下淋巴囊注射

1.颌下囊　2.胸囊　3.腹囊　4.股囊　5.胫囊　6.侧囊　7.头背囊

四、实验动物的取血方法

药理实验常需采集动物的血液标本用于生化分析等用途，采血技术决定了样本的质量优劣，对实验结果影响较大。不同动物、不同用途应采用不同的采血方法。

1.小鼠和大鼠

剪尾取血：将鼠固定在特制筒内，使鼠尾露在外面。剪掉鼠尾（小鼠1~2 mm；大鼠5~10 mm），用拇指和食指由尾根向尾尖挤按，血液即从尾尖流出。小鼠每次可采血0.1 ml，大鼠每次可采血0.5 ml。注意：只能剪去尾尖，如剪去过多组织，反而流血少。下次取血时，只需将尾尖血痂剪掉即可，适用于多次采血。

眼眶取血：左手持鼠，使眼球突出，并使头向下。右手持弯曲镊，钳夹一侧眼球根部，快速将眼球摘除。血液即可从断裂的眼眶动脉、静脉涌出，血量约为鼠体重的4%~5%，适用于一次性采大量血。

眼球后静脉丛取血：左手持鼠，使眼球突出，右手持一特制玻璃吸管，沿内眦眼眶后壁刺入，轻轻转动，血液自动进入吸管。得到所需血量后，拔出吸管，用干棉球轻按内眦片刻止血，适用于多次采少量血。

断头取血：左手固定动物头颈部向下倾，用利剪剪断鼠颈，血液自颈部流出滴入收集的容器。小鼠可取血约1 ml，大鼠可取血约8 ml。

2.豚鼠

心脏穿刺采血：将动物仰卧位固定，左手拇指在胸骨一侧，食指和中指于胸骨另一侧固定心脏，在心尖搏动最明显处将连有注射器的7号针头与胸壁垂直刺入胸腔，当持针手感到心脏搏动时，再稍刺入，即可见血液自心脏流进注射器，固定针头，抽出所需血量，拔出针头。注意取血时，针头宜直入直出，勿在胸腔内左右探索。一次可取血3~5 ml，但短时间内不宜再次取血，以免心脏损伤严重而致动物死亡。本法适用于较大量的取血。

3.家兔

耳缘静脉取血：拔去耳缘部被毛，用灯泡照射加热耳朵或以75%酒精涂擦局部，使静脉扩张。再用石蜡油涂擦耳缘，以防流出的血液凝固或散开不成滴。用粗针头逆静脉回流方向刺破静脉或用刀片切开静脉，血液可自动流出，一般可采血2~3 ml，取血后干棉球压迫止血。

耳中央动脉取血：左手固定兔耳，右手持注射器，在中央动脉末端向心方向刺入动脉，动脉血立即进入针筒，一次可取血15 ml。因耳中央动脉容易发生痉挛收缩，必须先让兔耳充分充血，并在痉挛前迅速完成抽血，抽血后干棉球压迫止血。

心脏取血：同豚鼠的心脏取血方法。

4.狗

头静脉和小隐静脉取血：固定动物，剪去局部被毛，碘酒消毒，使静脉充盈，常规穿刺即可抽出血液。必要时亦可从心脏、颈静脉、股动脉取血。

耳缘静脉取血：需少量血可采用此法。方法同家兔。

五、实验动物的麻醉方法

急性或慢性动物实验中，经常需要麻醉动物。麻醉剂可抑制中枢神经系统，还会引起其他生理功能的变化。因此，选择正确的麻醉剂及麻醉方式，对实验顺利进行以及良好的实验结果极为重要。根据实验目的、动物种类，可选择不同的麻醉剂和麻醉方法。

1.吸入麻醉

小鼠、大鼠常用乙醚吸入麻醉。将5~10 ml乙醚浸湿脱脂棉，放在玻璃容器底部，随即将动物放在容器的网状隔板上。盖上盖，约20~30秒动物进入麻醉状态。亦可将浸湿乙醚的棉球放入小烧杯中，扣在动物的口鼻部，让其吸入麻醉。

除了大鼠、小鼠，其他动物亦可采用乙醚麻醉，如狗、猫、兔等。乙醚麻醉量和致死量相差较大，安全度大。乙醚麻醉深度容易掌握，麻醉后恢复较快，适用于时间不长的手术。

2.注射麻醉

注射麻醉是最常用的麻醉方法。常用的药物有巴比妥类、乌拉坦和氯醛糖。可根据动物的特点、实验目的和手术过程选择药物。

巴比妥类对动物有良好的麻醉作用，手术时间较长者可选用苯巴比妥或戊巴比妥钠，若要动物术后恢复者宜用作用时间较短的戊巴比妥钠、硫喷妥钠。乌拉坦对动物的作用强而迅速，对大鼠和猫的血压有影响，可引起血压下降，呼吸中枢阈略微提高。氯醛糖可麻醉运动感觉脊髓中枢而不影响反射作用，增强肾上腺素兴奋子宫的作用，降低副交感神经的作用。

静脉麻醉时，剂量要准确，浓度要适中，注射速度要缓慢、均匀。冬季做实验时，应将药物加温到动物体温水平。注射麻醉剂后，密切观察动物眼睑、角膜及趾反射，避免麻醉过深引起动物死亡。一旦麻醉过量，尽早采取人工呼吸等措施。

药物的用法、用量及配制注意事项可参考附录三。

六、实验动物的安乐死方法

（1）蛙和蟾蜍　可采用断头安乐死，亦可用探针破坏大脑和脊髓安乐死。

（2）小鼠和大鼠　常采用颈椎脱臼法，即用左手拇指和食指将其头部紧按在硬的物体上，右手抓住鼠尾，并用力向后牵拉，使颈椎脱位，实现安乐死。

（3）兔、猫和狗　空气栓塞法：用50~100 ml注射器，往静脉内迅速注入空气，动物因血管气栓致死。兔和猫注射空气量为10~20 ml，狗为70~150 ml。

（4）麻醉致死法　注射致死剂量的麻醉药，如用2~3倍麻醉剂量的戊巴比妥钠静脉注射，使动物生命中枢受到严重抑制，实现安乐死。

（5）大量放血法　在麻醉状态下，切断颈动脉或股动脉，动物因大量失血实现安乐死。

七、动物实验外科基本操作技术

（一）组织切开、分离与止血

1.组织切开

组织切开的一般原则如下：

（1）根据实验目的及要求确定手术切口的部位和大小。如肾切除取左背部斜切口，肠切除取腹正中切口。

（2）根据不同部位的切口采用不同的执刀方法。常用的执刀方法有三种，如图1-2-17。

握持式（图1-2-17A）：全手握持刀柄，拇指与食指紧捏刀柄刻痕处，主要力量集中在手腕。用于切割范围广、用力较大的切口，如切开较长的皮肤切口、筋膜、慢性增生组织等。

执弓式（图1-2-17B）：是最常用的一种执刀方式，以手指按刀背后的三分之一处，力量来源于手腕与手指，主要用于切开皮肤腹膜及切断钳夹组织。

执笔式（图1-2-17C）：类似于执钢笔，主要力量分布在手指处，腕部做辅助，用于力量小、短距离的精细操作，例如切割短小切口，分离血管、神经等。

【注意事项】

（1）切开前，应先将切口部位的皮肤（或其他组织）拉紧，使其平坦紧绷而固定。

（2）刀刃与切开的组织垂直，以一次切开为佳。

（3）组织要逐层切开，并按皮肤纹理或各组织的纤维方向切开为佳。

（4）组织的切开处应选择无重要血管及神经横贯的地方，以免将其损伤。

（5）选择切口时，应注意选择易于敷料或导管包扎和固定的部位。避免术后动物活动时敷料被碰撞、摩擦而脱落。

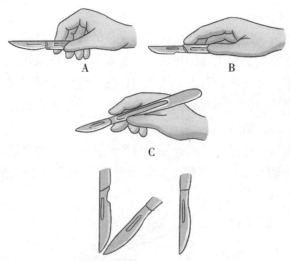

图 1-2-17 执刀方法和组织切开方法

A.握持式 B.执弓式 C.执笔式

2.组织分离

分离目的在于充分显露深层的组织或血管，便于手术操作。组织分离的一般原则如下：

（1）根据不同部位手术的需要采用不同的分离方法。常用的分离方法有两种：①用刀或剪作锐性分离，用剪割的方式将组织分离。该方法常用于致密组织，如皮肤、韧带、筋膜等组织的分离。②用止血钳、手指或刀柄等将组织推开或牵拉开作钝性分离。该方法多用于皮下组织、肌肉筋膜间隙等疏松组织的分离。

（2）沿正常组织间隙分离。这样易于分离，且出血少，视野干净、清楚。

【注意事项】

（1）肌肉的分离应顺肌纤维方向作钝性分离。若需要横行切断分离，应在切断处上下端先夹两把血管钳，切断后，结扎两处断端，以防止肌肉中血管出血。

（2）神经、血管的分离应顺其平行方向分离。要求动作轻柔，细心操作，不可粗暴，切忌横向过分拉扯，以防断裂。

3.止血

对组织切开、分离过程中所造成的出血必须及时止血。完善的止血不仅可以防止继续失血，还可以使术野清楚地显露，有利于手术的顺利进行。一般常用的止血方法有压迫止血法、钳夹止血法、结扎止血法、药物止血法、烧烙止血法等。

（1）压迫止血法 用灭菌纱布或棉球压迫出血部位，多适用于毛细血管渗血。止血时，将纱布或棉球用温热生理盐水打湿拧干后，按压在出血部位片刻即可，对于较大血管出血时可先用压迫止血法后再以其他方法止血。

（2）钳夹止血法 用血管钳的尖端垂直夹住出血血管端。小的血管出血经钳夹后，放松止血钳可不再出血。大的血管出血，应先用钳夹法后再用结扎法止血。

（3）结扎止血法　结扎止血法是常用且可靠的止血方法。结扎止血法又可分单纯结扎止血法和贯穿结扎两种。

单纯结扎止血法：用丝线绕过止血钳所夹住的血管及组织而结扎，适用于一般部位经压迫止血无效或较大血管出血的止血。出血点用纱布压迫蘸吸后，迅速用止血钳尖端逐个夹住血管断端，要夹准、夹牢。结扎时，先将止血钳尾竖起，将结扎线绕过钳夹点之下，再将钳放平后钳尖端稍翘起。打第一个结时，边扎紧边慢慢松开止血钳，完全扎紧后，再打第二个结，如图1-2-18。

贯穿结扎止血法：将结扎线用缝针穿过所钳夹组织（勿穿透血管壁）后结扎。常适用大血管出血。为防止结扎线滑脱，其常用方法有"8"字缝合结扎法和单纯贯穿结扎法两种，如图1-2-19。

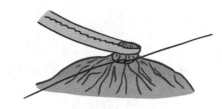

图1-2-18　单纯结扎止血法

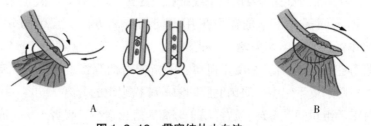

A　　　　　　　　　　　　　　　　　　　B

图1-2-19　贯穿结扎止血法

A. "8"字缝合结扎法　B. 单纯贯穿结扎法

（4）其他止血方法　药物止血法：用1%～2%麻黄碱或0.005%～0.01%肾上腺素液浸湿纱布或棉球，敷压出血处，使血管收缩而止血。

烧烙止血法：常用电凝器或电刀直接烧灼血管断裂处，使血液凝固而达到止血目的，常用于创口渗血和小血管出血。该方法止血快，切口内不留结扎线，有利于术后刀口恢复。

（二）缝合、打结

1. 缝合

常用的缝合种类包括间断缝合（结节缝合）、褥式缝合、"8"字缝合、连续缝合、毯边缝合、浆肌层单缝合、浆肌层双缝合、全层内翻缝合、荷包缝合。其缝合方法如下：

（1）间断缝合（结节缝合）　将缝线穿过切口两侧边缘即行打结。常用于皮肤、皮下组织、黏膜或筋膜的缝合，如图1-2-20。

（2）褥式缝合　为两个相反方向而接连的间断缝合，可使切口边缘外翻，有垂直及平行两种褥式缝合，如图1-2-21。常用于松弛部位皮肤的缝合或血管缝合。

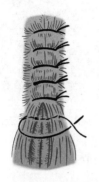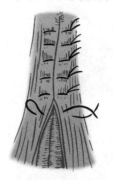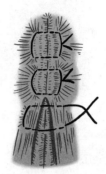

图1-2-20　间断缝合　　　　图1-2-21　褥式缝合（垂直、平行）

（3）"8"字缝合　为两个相反方向交叉的间断缝合组成，如图1-2-22。多用于筋膜或腱膜的缝合。

（4）连续缝合　于切口的一端开始，先做一间断缝合后不剪断线，用同一缝线作连续缝合至切口的另一端再行打结。在最后打结时，缝针穿出后线头应留在最后一个结节的另一边，作为打结依靠用。连续缝合常用于腹膜及胃肠道吻合口内层缝合，如图1-2-23。

（5）毯边缝合（连续锁边缝合）　缝合方法和连续缝合基本相似。但在缝合过程中每次将缝线交错固定，如图1-2-24，多用于胃肠手术吻合口后壁内层缝合。

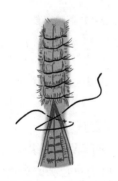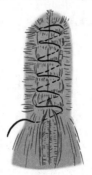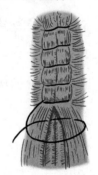

图1-2-22　"8"字缝合　　图1-2-23　连续缝合　　图1-2-24　毯边缝合

（6）浆肌层单缝合　缝线分别穿过切口两侧的浆膜及肌层即行打结，如图1-2-25。这样可使部分浆膜内翻对合。适用于胃肠道的外层缝合。

（7）浆肌层连续缝合　于切口的一端先做一浆肌层单缝合，再用同一缝线平行切口连续做浆肌层缝合至切口另一端，如图1-2-26。适用于胃肠道手术外层缝合。

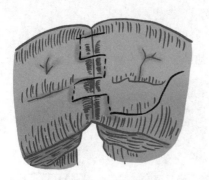
图 1-2-25 基浆层单缝合

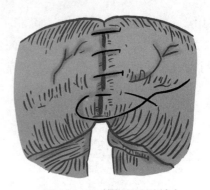
图 1-2-26 基浆层连续缝合

（8）全层内翻缝合　一侧黏膜进针和浆膜出针，线结打在腔内同时形成内翻，如图1-2-27。适用于胃肠道的前壁内层缝合。

（9）荷包缝合　即作环状的浆肌层连续缝合，如图1-2-28。常用于胃肠小的创口包埋使之内翻缝合。

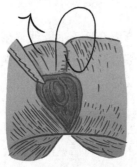
图 1-2-27 全层内翻缝合

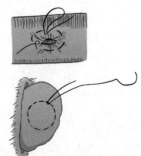
图 1-2-28 荷包缝合

【注意事项】

（1）缝合前，应彻底止血，并清除缝合口内的血凝块及游离组织，必要时加以冲洗。

（2）缝合时，缝针穿入或穿出组织应与该组织表面相垂直。

（3）入孔和出孔距皮肤切口边缘一般要0.5~1.0 cm，筋膜及其他组织约0.2~0.5 cm。

（4）两边针孔要对称，缝线不要过紧、过密，以切口能对合严密为度，有利切口边缘血液循环。

（5）深切口需按原解剖层次对合缝合。

（6）线结应位于切口的同一侧。

（7）缝合皮肤后，应用有齿镊对合切口，切勿使切口皮肤边沿内翻，影响切口愈合。

2.打结

正确而牢固地打结是结扎止血和缝合的重要环节，熟练地进行打结可缩短手术时间。正确的扣结种类包括方结、外科结、三重结，不正确的扣结有假结、滑结。假结、滑结是打结中最忌的，必须避免。如图1-2-29。

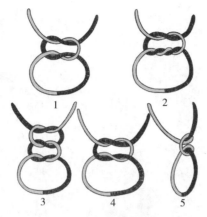

图 1-2-29　结的种类

1.方结　2.外科结　3.三重结　4.假结　5.滑结

（1）方结　用于一般结扎止血和各种缝合的结扎。结扎时两端必须用力均匀，避免形成滑结。

（2）外科结　结扎第一道时，两线重复交叉两圈，第二道线方法同方结。此种结因第一道结线绕两圈，摩擦面增大，不易松开。常用于结扎大血管。

（3）三重结　用于重要组织和大血管的结扎。在方结基础上再增加一道结扎。

常用的打结方法如下：

（1）单手打结法　适用于各部位的打结，操作简便，速度快。如图1-2-30。

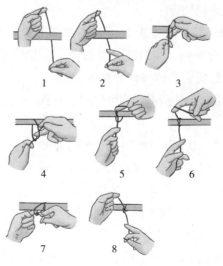

图 1-2-30　单手打结法

（2）止血钳打结法　用于浅部缝合的结扎、深部狭小术野的结扎及某些精细手术的结扎，如图1-2-31。

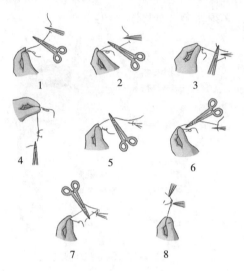

图1-2-31　止血钳打结法

（三）血管内插管

动物实验往往需反复采血、给药、补充电解质和营养液等，为此要采用血管内插管，即在动物某一血管内插入一定长度的尼龙或塑料导管从皮下引至体外，与体外实验装置管道相连接。血管内插管操作方便，易于固定，通道维持时间长。动物实验中血管内插管最常选用的血管是颈外静脉、颈总动脉、股静脉、股动脉，这些血管在体表分布较浅，管径比较大，容易辨认。

1. 颈外静脉和颈总动脉插管

犬、猪、兔、猫的颈外静脉很粗大，是头颈部的静脉主干，在颈部两侧皮下很浅部位。颈总动脉位于气管外侧，胸锁乳突肌前缘，其腹面被胸骨舌骨肌和胸骨甲状肌遮盖。颈外静脉和颈总动脉插管具体操作方法如下：

（1）手术区准备　将动物麻醉后，仰卧位固定于手术台上，头偏向另一侧，剪去插管侧部位的被毛，消毒、铺巾。

（2）颈外静脉和颈总动脉分离　在气管的外侧、胸骨切迹至甲状软骨连线的中点，向两端切开皮肤，用手指在皮肤外面向上顶起，即可见到呈暗紫色的粗大血管——颈外静脉，将静脉周围的皮下组织轻轻钝性分离一段即可插管，如图1-2-32。

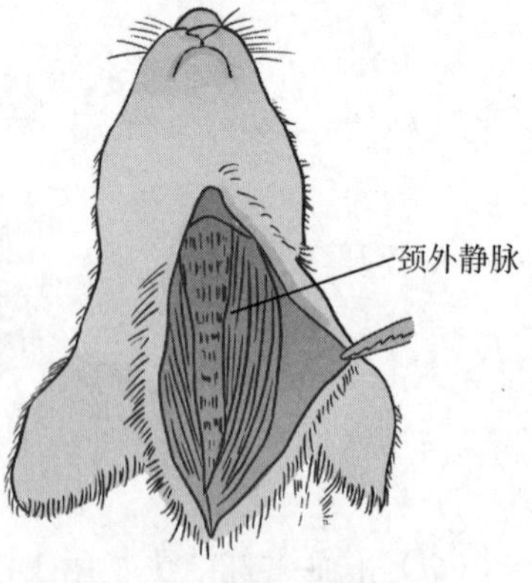

沿胸锁乳突肌前缘分离胸骨舌骨肌与胸骨甲状肌之间的结缔组织，在肌缝下找到呈粉红色的较粗血管，用手指触之有搏动感，即为颈总动脉。分离颈总动脉时应选在距甲状腺以下较远地方开始，防止将甲状腺

颈外静脉

图1-2-32　家兔颈外静脉分离

前动脉切断，用眼科镊轻轻钝性分离该动脉与神经之间的结缔组织，切勿损伤血管和神经。在分离过程中，应不时地以生理盐水湿润手术切口组织，并用纱布擦拭血液；为了便于动脉插管，颈总动脉应尽量分离得长一些。一般犬和小型猪分离5~6 cm，家兔和猫4~5 cm，豚鼠和大鼠2~3 cm。

（3）颈外静脉和颈总动脉内置管　先准备好导管，从插入端剪一斜面，另一端连接于装有抗凝溶液或生理盐水的注射针或输液装置上，让导管内充满溶液，然后在分离好的静脉或动脉下面穿过两根结扎线，一根先在远心端结扎后，用手轻轻提起结扎线，将动脉或静脉向前牵拉，让其有一定的张力，用眼科剪在离结扎线的下方血管壁上剪一"V"形小口，轻轻地将准备好的导管从小口插入，将近心端的一根结扎线于插入口的下方绑扎，将血管壁紧紧扎于导管四周，再用结扎的线固定导管，防止导管滑脱，导管固定好后，将动脉或静脉放回原位，试向血管内输入生理盐水，观察其是否通畅和是否有溶液漏出。如有凝血，需加压冲洗。如有漏出，则应重新结扎近心端结扎处，此时根据实验需要，可以关闭缝合切口，将插入导管一端留到体外，连接到输液装置上。

附：小鼠主要脏器的解剖位置与形态特征

（1）肺　小鼠肺分左右两叶，右肺分为四叶（尖叶、心叶、膈叶、副叶），左肺为一整叶。左肺有一条不太深的沟，将其分成两段，似不完全的整叶，如图1-2-33。

（2）心脏　小鼠心脏呈圆锥状，位于近胸骨端，心尖位于第四肋间。小鼠心耳较大。小鼠的心脏及主要血管，如图1-2-34。

（3）肝　小鼠肝脏附于膈上，呈暗褐色，分为五叶（外侧左叶、内侧左叶、外侧右叶、内侧右叶、尾状叶）。如图1-2-35。

（4）胃　胃分贲门、幽门、胃底及胃体。幽门内壁黏膜呈皱褶状。如图1-2-36。

（5）肠　肠分小肠与大肠，小肠包括十二指肠、空肠和回肠，小鼠小肠长约50~65 cm。大肠分盲肠、结肠、直肠，大肠长约12~17 cm。

（6）脾　脾斜卧于胃的左侧，呈暗红色，长条扁平状。

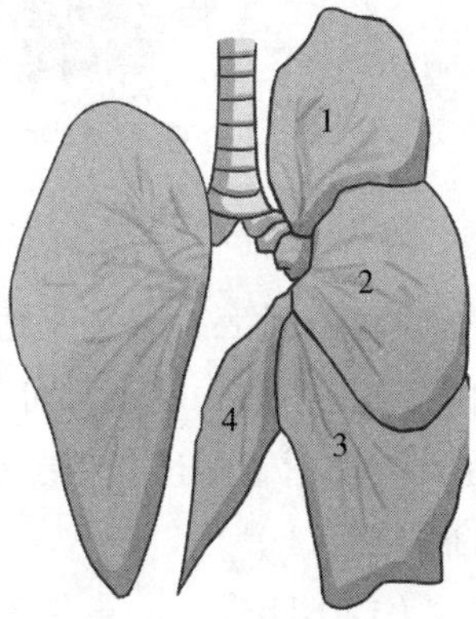

（7）胰　胰脏在十二指肠附近，呈粉红色。小鼠胰脏及胆总管十二指肠开口如图1-2-37。

图1-2-33　小鼠肺
1.尖叶　2.心叶　3.膈叶　4.副叶

（8）肾　肾脏在腹腔的背壁，为一对形如蚕豆、呈暗红色的脏器，右肾比左肾位置稍高，肾脏的前方有肾上腺，每肾内侧各有一条输尿管，开口于膀胱的背侧。

（9）膀胱　膀胱位于腹腔的后端，直通于尿道口。

（10）睾丸　小鼠睾丸有一对，幼年时的睾丸位于腹腔内，性成熟以后则下降到阴囊内。成年小鼠睾丸体积为8.5 mm×5 mm×5 mm，重量70~90 mg。睾丸表面为纤维性结缔组织，内部有无数曲精细管产生精子，间质组织产生雄性激素。

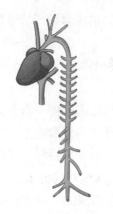

图1-2-34　小鼠的心脏及主要血管

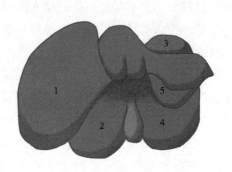

图1-2-35　小鼠肝脏

1.左外侧叶　2.左内侧叶　3.右外侧叶　4.右内侧叶　5.尾状叶

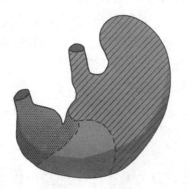

图1-2-36　小鼠胃

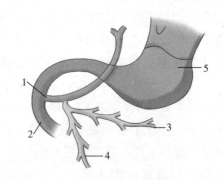

图1-2-37　小鼠胰脏及胆总管十二指肠开口

1.胆总管　2.十二指肠　3.前大胰腺管　4.后大胰腺管　5.胃

（11）附睾　附睾是由许多弯曲相通的细管组成，是接受并暂时贮藏精子的地方。附睾分头、体、尾三部分。附睾头部与睾丸上部的精细管连接，体部在睾丸一侧下行，尾部与输精管相连。精子在通过附睾期间成熟。成熟的有受精力的精子通过与附睾相接的输精管。

（12）卵巢　卵巢是产生卵子的地方。形似绿豆状，粉红色，左右各一，位于肾脏下方。成年小鼠除妊娠期以外，通常全年呈周期性（4~5日）排卵。

（13）子宫　小鼠为双角子宫。子宫为Y字形，分子宫角、子宫体。子宫角始于输卵管结合部，沿体背面下行，左右子宫角在膀胱背面会合，形成子宫体。小鼠子宫体分前后两部，前部由中隔分开，左右成对，形成两个单独的子宫，后部中隔消失，左右子宫会合后逐渐形成子宫颈，子宫颈末端突出于阴道，形如小丘。

（14）阴道　阴道前部连接子宫。

（15）输精管　输精管是精子通过的管道。由附睾尾部引出的毛细管，在精囊腺下面、膀胱的背侧汇合进入尿道。成年小鼠的输精管内存有无数的有受精能力的精子。

（16）输卵管　输卵管是卵子受精及通过的管道。输卵管呈弯曲状，左右各一条，位于卵巢与子宫角之间，前端似喇叭口，开口朝向卵巢，后端紧接于子宫。

Section 3　Dosage Calculation in Animal Experiments

~ ~ . ~ . ~ . ~ . ~ . ~ . ~ . ~ . ~ . ~ . ~ . ~ . ~ . ~ . ~ . ~ . ~ . ~ . ~ . ~

Knowledge

1. Calculation methods among dosage, drug concentration and administration volume.
2. Conversion rules of dosage among lab animals.
3. Methods of describing drug concentration.
4. Methods to determine the administration volume in animal experiments.

Skill

1. Accurately figure out the dosage, drug concentration and administration volume according to the study design.
2. Determine the appropriate dosage according to the experiment purpose.

~ ~ . ~ . ~ . ~ . ~ . ~ . ~ . ~ . ~ . ~ . ~ . ~ . ~ . ~ . ~ . ~ . ~ . ~ . ~ . ~

Dosage Determination

In pharmacology experiments, the common unit for dose is 'mg/kg', referring to the mass (mg) of drugs that used on per unit weight (kg) of animals.The administration dose is based on practical experiences. According to the experiment design, you may refer to similar previous studies, in order to find an appropriate dosage. In case there's no useful data, you can refer to some similar drugs. You may also try 1/5 to 1/3 of the studied drug's lethal dose (LD_{50}).

Dose conversions among lab animals are based on the ratio of body surface per unit body weight. This conversion may not be very accurate, therefore you should always double-check its results.

Calculation of Drug Concentration and Administration Volume

1. Descriptions of Drug Concentration

1.1 Mass concentration

The commonly-used unit in describing the mass concentration a drug solution is 'g/L'or percentage concentration (%). For example, when preparing the 9.0 g/L or normal (0.9%) saline, you can dissolve 9.0 g of sodium chloride in some distilled water, and dilute it to 1000 ml also with distilled water, then stir well.

1.2 Amount of substance concentration

The amount of substance concentration is commonly described with the unit of 'mol/L' or 'mmol/L'. For example, to prepare a beaker of 1.83×10^{-2} mmol/L procaine hydrochloride solution, as the molecular weight of this compound is 272.8, you can dissolve 4.99 g of procaine hydrochloride, then dilute it to 1000ml and stir well.

2. Calculation of Administration Volume

The dosage in pharmacology experiments is generally described with the unit of 'mg/kg'. However, we often use 'mg/10g' on mice and toads, and 'mg/100g' on rats and guinea pigs. Conversions between the dosage and administration volume are required with methods below.

2.1 To calculate the administration volume based on a known drug concentration and its dosage, the formula is illustrated below:

$$\text{Administration Volume (ml)} = \frac{\text{Dosage (mg/kg)} \times \text{Body Weight (kg)}}{\text{Drug Concentration (mg/ml)}}$$

For example, as the dose of morphine hydrochloride for intraperitoneal injection on mice is 10 mg/kg, how many millilitres of 1 g/L morphine hydrochloride solution will be injected into a 22g mouse?

$$\text{Calculation: Administration Volume (ml)} = \frac{10 \text{ mg/kg} \times 0.022 \text{ kg}}{1 \text{ mg/ml}} = 0.22 \text{ ml}$$

You may convert the dose unit into 'ml/10g' as it's more convenient.

Other Calculation Processes:

Concentration of Morphine Hydrochloride: 1 g/L → 1 mg/ml

Dosage: 10 mg/kg → 0.1 mg/10 g → 0.1 ml/10g

Administration Volume = 0.1 ml ÷ 10 g × 22 g = 0.22 ml

2.2 To calculate the concentration (g/L) of required solutions according to the dose and administration volume, the formula is illustrated below:

$$\text{Solution Concentration (g/L)} = \frac{\text{Dosage (g/kg)}}{\text{Administration Volume (L/kg)}}$$

For example: what's the concentration of the morphine hydrochloride solution, as its dosage for subcutaneous injection on rabbits is 10 mg/kg, and the maximum dosing volume of it is 1 ml/kg.

$$\text{Calculation: Solution Concentration (g/L)} = \frac{0.01 \text{ (g/kg)}}{0.001 \text{ (L/kg)}} = 10 \text{g/L}$$

You may also solve similar tasks according to the following ideas:

As 1 ml of the solution contains 10 mg of morphine hydrochloride, while injecting it to the rabbit at a dose of 10 mg/kg with the 1 ml/kg solution.

$$1 : 10 = 1000 : X$$
$$X = 10000 \text{ mg} = 10 \text{ g}$$

Hence, concentration of the morphine hydrochloride solution to be prepared is 10 g/L.

2.3 We've found the most appropriate administration volume and dose routes for some specific animals(Appendix 2). When formulate drugs for them, we should refer to these records.

For example, providing an appropriate concentration for injecting a certain drug into the rat's intraperitoneal cavity at a dose of 25 mg/kg.

Calculation: according Appendix 2, the appropriate dose for intraperitoneal injection on rats ranged from 0.5 to 1 ml/100 g. Assuming the dosing volume is 0.5 ml/100g, its concentration can be figured out with the process below:

$$C = \frac{\text{Dose}}{\text{Volume}} = \frac{25\text{mg/kg}}{0.5\text{ml/100g}} = \frac{25\text{mg/1000g}}{0.5\text{ml/100g}} = 5 \text{ mg/ml} = 0.5\%$$

Hence, we should formulate the drug at a concentration of 5 mg/ml (0.5%), which means there are 0.5 g drugs in per 100ml of the solution.

3. Dosage Conversion among Commonly-Used Lab Animals

The equivalent dose of a certain drug for different animals may greatly vary if you calculate it with body weight (mg/kg), however it can would be more accurate if been calculated with body surface area (mg/m^2). To sum up, it's more practical to convert the dosage among animals according to their body surface area.

$$\text{Body surface Area （m}^2） = \frac{K \times W^{2/3}}{10000}$$

K: a constant, W: body weight (g)

It is more convenient to solve such tasks with 'factors of mg/kg-mg/m^2 conversion' or the ratio of body surface area per body weight (Appendix 1).

For example, estimating the gavage dosage of a certain drug on a 10 kg dog, which is at a dose of 250 mg/kg on rats.

3.1 Direct calculation with the body surface area formula

Step 1: calculation of rat's body surface area.

$$\text{Rat's Body Surface Area} = \frac{9.1 \times 200^{2/3}}{10000} = 0.0311 \text{m}^2$$

Step 2: convert 250 mg/kg into X mg/m^2.

$$\text{Rat's Dosage according to the Body Surface Area} = \frac{250 \times 0.2}{0.0311} = 1068 \text{ mg/m}^2$$

Step 3: calculation of dog's body surface area.

$$\text{Body Surface Area of a 10 kg Dog} = \frac{11.2 \times 10000^{2/3}}{10000} = 0.5198 \text{ m}^2$$

Step 4: calculation of dog's dosage.

$$\text{Dog's Dosage} = \frac{1068 \times 0.5198}{10} = 84 \text{ mg/kg}$$

3.2 Calculation with 'factors of mg/kg-mg/m² conversion'

$$\text{Dog's Dosage} = \frac{250 \times 6 \text{ (Rat's Conversion Factor)}}{19 \text{ (Dog's Conversion Factor)}} = 79 \text{ mg/kg}$$

3.3 Calculation with 'the ratio of body surface area per body weight'

$$\text{Dog's Dosage} = \frac{250 \times 0.16 \text{ (Dog's Ratio)}}{0.47 \text{ (Rat's Ratio)}} = 85 \text{ mg/kg}$$

Homework

1. For a certain drug with an intraperitoneal dosage of 10 mg/kg and a 0.1 ml/10 g administration volume on mice, what's the concentration and how much millilitres of this solution should be injected into a 25 g mouse?

2. An experiment design is described as follows: 30 mice are equally divided into 3 groups, and receive intraperitoneal injections of a certain drug at different dosages as listed 30 mg/kg, 60 mg/kg and 120 mg/kg. As the original concentration of this drug is 1.5%, how would you formulate the drug for this study? Figure out an appropriate administration volume and state a suitable total volume of the solution.

3. Convert the gavage dose of 100 mg/kg on rats to human oral dose.

第三章　动物实验给药量的计算

知识要求

1.掌握药物剂量、浓度、给药容量之间的换算方法，动物之间剂量换算关系。

2.熟悉药物浓度表示方法，动物给药剂量确定方法。

能力要求

1.根据实验设计熟练计算给药剂量、药物浓度和给药容量。

2.根据实验设计确定合适的给药剂量。

一、给药剂量的确定

药理实验中给予动物的药物剂量单位是mg/kg，定义为动物单位体重（kg）所用药物的质量（mg）。给药剂量来自于实践经验，非凭空想象而来。根据具体情况，我们可以查阅文献资料，参考前人的经验，如实验目的、方法类似，可采用文献中的药物剂量。有时查不到合适的剂量，或者所用药物无前人经验，可以参考类似药物或者致死量LD_{50}，可以采用1/5~1/3的致死量。

不同种属动物之间的剂量换算，不是通过体重比例来增减，而需通过单位体重所占体表面积的比值来换算。换算的剂量可能有所偏差，一般作为参考值。

二、药物浓度及给药容量的计算

（一）药理实验常用药物浓度表示方法

1.质量浓度　常用单位为或g/L或百分比浓度（%）。如配制9.0 g/L或（0.9%）生理盐水，应将9.0 g氯化钠用少量蒸馏水溶解后，再加蒸馏水至1000 ml，搅拌均匀，即得。

2.物质的量浓度　常用单位为mol/L或mmol/L。如配制1.83×10^{-2} mmol/L盐酸普鲁卡因溶液时，将4.99 g盐酸普鲁卡因用少量蒸馏水溶解后，再加水至1000 ml，摇匀，即得（盐酸普鲁卡因的分子量为272.8）。

（二）动物给药容量的换算

实验动物用药剂量，一般用mg/kg体重表示，但小鼠和蟾蜍用mg/10g体重表示，大鼠和豚鼠用mg/100g体重表示。有以下三种情况，需要进行换算：

（1）根据已知药物浓度和给药剂量计算给药容量，计算公式如下：

$$给药容量（ml）= \frac{剂量（mg/kg）\times 动物体重（kg）}{药液浓度（mg/ml）}$$

举例：盐酸吗啡溶液浓度为1 g/L，小鼠腹腔注射剂量为10 mg/kg体重，小鼠体重22 g，应给小鼠注射多少毫升？

计算过程：给药容量（ml）= $\dfrac{10 \text{ mg/kg} \times 0.022 \text{ kg}}{1 \text{ mg/ml}}$ =0.22 ml

在实际工作中，剂量单位改写成mg/10 g，由浓度推算成ml/10 g更方便。

推算过程如下：

盐酸吗啡浓度：1 g/L→1 mg/ml；

注射剂量：10 mg/kg→0.1 mg/10g→0.1 ml/10g；

注射容量＝0.1ml÷10 g×22 g=0.22 ml

（2）根据药物剂量和设定的给药容量，计算应配制的药液浓度（g/L），计算公式如下：

$$药液浓度（g/L）= \frac{给药剂量（g/kg）}{给药容量（L/kg）}$$

举例：兔皮下注射盐酸吗啡剂量为10 mg/kg，最大注射容量为1ml/kg，应配制的药液浓度是多少？

代入上述公式,

$$药液浓度（g/L）= \frac{0.01（g/kg）}{0.001（L/kg）} = 10 \text{ g/L}$$

在实际工作中,亦可按下面思路推算:

按剂量10 mg/kg相当于容量1 ml/kg注射时,1 ml药液应含10 mg盐酸吗啡。

$$1:10 = 1000:X$$

$$X = 10000 \text{ mg} = 10 \text{ g}$$

即应配制盐酸吗啡溶液浓度为10 g/L。

（3）特定动物、特定给药途径有最适宜的给药容量（见附录二）,应选适宜的给药容量来配制药物。

举例:某药物经大鼠腹腔注射,剂量为25 mg/kg。问:配制何种浓度较为适宜?

解:大鼠腹腔注射的适宜剂量是0.5~1 ml/100 g（见附录二）,假设选择给药容量为0.5 ml/100 g,已知剂量为25 mg/kg,则药物浓度计算如下:

$$C = \frac{给药剂量}{给药容量} = \frac{25 \text{ mg/kg}}{0.5 \text{ ml/100 g}} = \frac{25 \text{ mg/1000 g}}{0.5 \text{ ml/100 g}} = 5 \text{ mg/ml} = 0.5\%$$

所以,配制药物浓度为5 mg/ml,换算为百分比浓度则为0.5%,即每100 ml溶液中含有药物的质量为0.5 g。

（三）常用动物之间的用药剂量换算

同一药物不同种属动物的等效剂量,如按mg/kg体重计算差异很大,而按体表面积计算,则很接近。也就是说动物的给药剂量按体表面积进行换算更切合实际。

$$动物体表面积（m^2） = \frac{K \times W^{2/3}}{10000}$$

式中,K为常数;W为体重（g）。

在实际工作中,用"mg/kg-mg/m²转换因子"或"每公斤体重占有体表面积的比值"计算更方便（转换参数见附录一）。

举例:某药给200 g大鼠的灌胃剂量250 mg/kg,试估计该药给10 kg狗灌胃时,应用多大剂量?

（1）应用体表面积公式直接计算

第1步:大鼠体表面积= $\frac{9.1 \times 200^{2/3}}{10000}$ =0.0311 m²

第2步:250 mg/kg改用mg/m²表示

$$大鼠按体表面积给药剂量 = \frac{250 \times 0.2}{0.0311} = 1068 \text{ mg/m}^2$$

第3步:10 kg狗的体表面积= $\frac{11.2 \times 10000^{2/3}}{10000}$ = 0.5198 m²

第4步：狗的给药剂量 $= \dfrac{1068 \times 0.5198}{10} = 84 \text{ mg/kg}$

（2）应用"mg/kg –mg/m² 转换因子"计算

$$狗的给药剂量 = \dfrac{250 \times 6 （大鼠转换因子）}{19 （狗转换因子）} = 79 \text{ mg/kg}$$

（3）用"占有体表面积比值"计算

$$狗的给药剂量 = \dfrac{250 \times 0.16 （狗体表面积比值）}{0.47 （大鼠体表面积比值）} = 85 \text{ mg/kg}$$

思考题

1.小鼠腹腔注射某药物，给药剂量为 10 mg/kg，给药容量为 0.1 ml/10 g，请问给 25 g 体重的小鼠注射应配制多少浓度、多少体积的药物溶液？

2.某实验设计如下：小鼠 30 只，平均分为三组，分别腹腔注射不同剂量某药物，具体为 30 mg/kg、60 mg/kg、120 mg/kg，已知该药物原浓度为 1.5%，请问如何配制药物用于完成实验？（解题时请结合给药途径选定适宜给药容量，并根据动物数配制合适体积的药物供使用）

3.某药物的大鼠灌胃给药剂量为 100mg/kg，试推算该药物的人口服剂量是多少？

Section 4   Basic Principles in Designing Pharmacology Experiments

Knowledge

1. Basic principles in designing pharmacology experiments.
2. Keypoints in designing pharmacology experiments.

Skill

1. Design pharmacology experiments with three basic principles.
2. Understand how to design the framework of a pharmacology experiment.

Pharmacology researches aim at revealing the effect of drugs, and the mechanism in these processes. As the study object in pharmacology researches are organisms, which have individual differences, the stability, repeatability and accuracy of study results may be affected. Therefore, to obtain credible results in pharmacology experiments, we must design the study scientifically. It may even ameliorate the result and simplify the work. Furthermore, we can get reliable and convincing experimental conclusions only when we follow the scientific experimental design, carry out correct operations, and cooperate with reasonable result analysis.

Basic Principles in Designing Pharmacology Experiments

Three major principles in designing pharmacology experiment are listed as follows: replication, randomisation and control.

1. Replication

Replication refers to good reproducibility and sufficient repetitions of an experiment. Because of the individual difference and experiment errors, it is difficult to come up with universal conclusions based on results of a single experiment on a small sample. However, when a same result, which fluctuates within an appropriate range, repeats for multiple times in a series of studies, the conclusion of these experiments tends to be reliable.

1.1 Sample size

The principle of replication is partially illustrated in the sample size of each group.

Generally, the larger the sample size is, the more accurate the study result will be. However, it is not economy and may greatly increase the cost. Besides, when studies already have good reproducibility, if we can not upgrade the accuracy of their P values, the more repeats within an experiment, the less valuable it is, because it indicates a huge fluctuation of experimental errors or results of them are very similar. Therefore, there is a certain limit in achieving the principle of replication by enlarging the sample size.

Sample size of experiments can be comprehensively considered according to factors below:

（1）The sample size of pharmacodynamic studies can be reduced if the tested drug has strong effect. Otherwise, you can select large sample size for weak effect drugs.

（2）Biological differences larger variation coefficient, smaller credibility limit and stricter P value range require larger sample size. On the contrary, it requires smaller sample size.

Generally, according to the size of animals in experiments, the sample size should not be less than the 'basic scale'.

Small Animals (mice, rats, fish, frogs): 10 cases per group for qualitative studies, and 30 cases per group for quantitative studies.

Medium animal (rabbits, guinea pigs): 6 cases per group for qualitative studies, and 20 cases per group for quantitative studies.

Large animals (dogs, cats, monkeys): 5 cases per group for qualitative studies, and 10 cases per group for quantitative studies.

1.2 Controlling interference factors

Besides the sample size, some relevant factors should also be controlled to reduce the interference. Otherwise, the obtained result may not be credible enough.

Relevant factors include as follows:

（1）Animals: strain, weight, sex, age, food, living environment, etc.

（2）Measuring instruments: precision, sensitivity, etc.

（3）Drug: batch number, purity, dosage, solvent, etc.

（4）Experimenter: proficiency, accuracy of judgment, etc.

2. Randomisation

Randomisation means that each object has the same chance of receiving treatments in an experiment, such as sampling, grouping, medication and testing, etc. This principle aims at reducing the interference or bias from subjective factors of the experimenter, in order to make the result more representative.

Usually, animals are randomly grouped in experiments according to the complete randomisation method, the balanced randomisation method or the balanced and ordered randomisation method.

2.1 Complete randomisation

It's also known as 'simple randomisation', which means all research objects are allocated to different treatment groups completely with a random number table or other randomisation methods. Whereas, we seldom apply this method in pharmacology experiments as it does not account the gender, age, weight, etc., of objects in study design, and it may interfere the result.

2.2 Balanced randomisation

It's also known as 'stratified randomisation', in which we employ some factors that are easy-to-control but may have great impacts on the result, such as gender, weight, etc., as stratified indicators, to balance each treatment group.

For example, at the beginning of an experiment, when animals have not received any treatments, their weight is usually an important factor that may affect the study result. You can randomly group them according to their body weight and keep the average weight of each group similar. This method is common in pharmacology experiments.

2.3 Balanced and ordered randomisation

This method is mainly employed in clinical practice or grouping animal pathological models. We usually balance the group first according to the gender, age, disease condition, etc., then randomly group the animal in a certain order. For example, we induce pathological models on animals first in some pharmacology experiments, then randomise them according to the body weight and disease conditions, keeping the body weight and disease condition of each group balanced.

3. Control

The principle of control: there are many factors that may affect the result of biological science studies, however only some of them are controllable. In order to deal with this problem, we can set up some control groups. A control group refers to the group that established for comparisons. There should be only one variable between each group in an experiment, whereas other factors should be kept unchanged to eliminate or reduce the influence from non-treatment factors. During the experiment, you should apply same operations to animal in parallel groups simultaneously in the same lab as much as possible, or the control may turn in vain. You may also observe the change of a certain index before and after the treatments on a single individual, as a self-control. You may also set up several parallel groups to discover the differences among groups, as the inter-group control. Common control group methods are listed below:

3.1 Negative control

In pharmacology experiments, animals in the negative control group receive no research-related treatments, providing negative results. Negative control also includes as follows:

Blank control is a control group without any treatment, which is usually applied in animal experiments to evaluate the accuracy of measurement methods and to detect whether the experiment is in normal state.

Sham control means animals in the sham control group receive the same treatment as those in the experimental group, however their drugs are replaced with solvent at the same dosage. Comparing the result of other groups with those of this group, you can find the effect of treatments in the study.

3.2 Positive control

Using a typical drug with definite curative effect as the control, producing a positive result, to verify the validity of the experiment. Study results of the positive control group should be positive, or the experiment may be invalid and you must check what's gone wrong in the study. Positive control also includes as follows:

Standard Control is using a standard or typical drug as the control, then evaluate the effect of experimental drugs by comparison.

Weak-Positive Control is in case of no suitable positive control drug, or to compare the mechanism of drugs, you can select some drugs with definite but not strong curative effect as the control.

3.3 Self control

Record the index of a same individual before and after treatment, then figure out the difference between them, or compare the result with that of untreated symmetrical parts. During this process, other factors should kept unchanged, making the observation index stable.

3.4 History control

Compare the study result with previous data that obtained in the same lab. This method can also be applied in quality control of laboratories.

Keypoints in Designing Pharmacology Experiments

You should also notice these key points when designing pharmacology experiments, in addition to three basic principles as follows:

（1）Clarify the study purpose: design experiments according to the task to be solved.

（2）Understand the research status: discover the research status referring to paper and literatures, to gain some ideas and references for your own experiment.

（3）Determine the experiment method and indicators for observation: select appropriate animal models or in vitro models based on your experiment design, following the principle of randomisation, control and replication. The observation indicator should be objective, reliable and comprehensive.

4. Dosage Determination

4.1 Dosage conversion

Convert the dosage among animals based on the body surface area, not the body weight.

4.2 Dosage selection

The dosage should be safe, otherwise it may make the experiment invalid. It's rational to set 3 or more dosage groups in a study to observe the dose-effect relationship.When studying new drugs, you may refer to its LD_{50}, and use 1/5 or 1/10 of it as the study dosage, keeping its therapeutic index above 3. When study the optimal dosage of a new drug, start the experiment on small animals, then increase the dose by 2 or 3.16 ($\sqrt{10}$) times in other animals. You may also increase it by 3 or 10 times in in-vitro experiments.

5. Determination of the Administration Route and Dosage Form

The administration route of drug should be as convenient as possible due to its nature. At least 2 routes of administration, oral administration and intraperitoneal or intravenous injection, should be studied in new drug researches.

The selection of dosage form is affected by the solubility of drugs. For example, drugs with good water-solubility can be made into solutions for oral administration or injection, and oil-soluble drugs may be made into emulsions for oral administration or intramuscular and intraperitoneal injection. Besides, drugs with poor solubility in both water and oil can be made into suspensions for oral administration.

6. Determining the Format of Experiment Records

Experiment records generally include these contents below:

（1）Title of the experiment.

（2）Participants.

（3）Samples include animal species, strains, weight, gender, etc., in animal experiments; name of the cell, the way of obtaining, etc., in cell experiments.

（4）Drugs include name, source, batch number, purity, dosage form, preparation method, etc. If the drug is a self-made compound, you should also state its quality control standard, ensuring its equivalent in each experiment.

（5）Environment includes time, room temperature, humidity, etc.

（6）Methods and procedures.

（7）Result and its format include design the original record table in advance, which is conducive to the data processing.

（8）Data processing method includes adopt suitable data management and analysis methods on different experiments to ensure correct conclusions.

第四章　药理学实验设计基本原则

知识要求

1.掌握药理学实验设计的基本原则。

2.熟悉药理学实验设计要点。

能力要求

1.在药理实验中能正确、熟练将三个基本原则运用其中。

2.对药理实验设计框架有初步的概念。

药理学研究的目的是揭示药物对机体的作用及规律，即药物有什么作用（或毒性），作用（或毒性）机制是什么。由于药理实验研究的对象是生物体，个体之间具有差异性，此差异是影响实验结果稳定性、重复性、准确性的重要因素。因此，要想得到可信的药理学实验结果，科学设计实验必不可少。依靠良好的实验设计，我们可以得到事半功倍的效果。只有遵循合理科学的实验设计，进行正确的实验操作，再配合合理的结果分析，这样才能获得可靠、令人信服的实验结论。

一、药理学实验设计的基本原则

药理学实验设计的三大原则是：重复、随机、对照。

（一）重复

重复的定义是：实验具有良好的重现性和有足够的重复数。由于生物个体的差异性和实验误差，仅根据一次实验或一个样本动物所得结果，往往很难下结论。在适当的范围内，多次重复得到同样的结果，说明此实验结论是可靠的。

1.样本量

重复的原则可通过实验各组的样本量来体现。通常样本量越大，实验结果越接近真实值。然而，这增加了人力、物力、财力，不符合经济原则。在良好的重现性前提下，如果统计 P 值相同，重复数越多的实验，价值越小。这说明实验误差波动太大或者两者均数相差太小。因此，单靠增加例数实现重复性是有一定限度的。

实验样本量的大小可根据以下几个因素综合考虑：①药效，药效作用强，样本数可减少，药效作用弱，可相应增大样本数。②生物差异，变异系数大则样本数大；可信限要求小，则样本数增加；P 值要求小，须加大样本数。

一般情况下，根据实验设计所采用的动物大小，应选择不少于"基本例数"的动物数进行实验。

小动物（小鼠、大鼠、鱼、蛙）：计量资料每组10例，计数资料每组30例。

中动物（兔或豚鼠）：计量资料每组6例，计数资料每组20例。

大动物（犬、猫或猴）：计量资料每组5例，计数资料每组10例。

2.干扰因素的控制

除了对动物样本量的设定外，实验过程还应控制影响实验结果的相关因素，只有减少无关因素的干扰，才可能得到客观、可信的结果。

相关控制因素包括：

（1）动物的品系、体重、性别、年龄、饲料、生活环境等。

（2）测定仪器的精密度、灵敏度等。

（3）药物的批号、纯度、剂量、溶剂等。

（4）实验者的操作水平、熟练程度、对指标判断准确程度等。

（二）随机

随机原则：随机是指在实验中，每个实验对象接受处理（抽样、分组、用药、检测等）时都具有同等机会。随机的目的是减少实验者主观因素的干扰，避免偏性误差，使样本具有更好的代表性。

在进行药理学动物实验时，实验动物分组通常需随机分组，随机分组主要采用完全随机、均衡随机和均衡顺序随机。

（1）完全随机　又称单纯随机，即所有研究对象完全按照随机原则（通过随机数字表或抽签的方式）分配到不同的处理组。该分组法一般在药理实验中很少采用，因为本法对实验对象的性别、年龄、体重、病情等均不做考虑，对所得结果难以判断、难以解释。

（2）均衡随机　又称分层随机，即将易于控制的、对实验结果可能影响较大的非处理因素作为分层指标，如：性别、体重等，人为地使各组在这些指标上达到均衡一致。例如：实验初始，实验动物还未接受任何处理，体重通常是影响实验的重要因素，可以根据体重均衡随机分组，分组后各组实验动物平均体重应接近。该法是药理学实验常用的分组方法。

（3）均衡顺序随机　该法主要用于临床或动物病理模型的抽样分组。即根据性别、年龄、病情等重要性进行均衡处理，再按照一定顺序随机分组。如：药理学实验中，动物需要先造成某一病理模型，然后再分组给药。实验模型造好后，根据主要因素，即疾病的病情（选择相应指标来判断）均衡分层表，再结合动物的体重进行随机分组，最终使各组动物病情、体重基本达到均衡，分组后对这些因素分析，各组之间不应有较大偏差。

（三）对照

对照原则：在生物科学实验中，影响实验的因素颇多，这些实验因素有些能控制，有些不能控制。为了解决这个问题，需设立对照组。对照组即在实验时设立的用于对比的组别，各实验组中除了一个变量改变，其他变量都相同，以此消除或减少非处理因素对实验结果的影响。在实验过程中注意要"同时、同地、同条件、同操作"，所有过程都要平行，否则失去对照的意义。对照时可在同一个体上观察给药前后或对称给药部位某指标变化，此为自身对照；也可设立若干平行组，观察不同组别之间指标的变化，此为组间对照。常用的对照方法有以下几种。

（1）阴性对照　在药理学实验中，主要针对实验预期结果而言，阴性对照组不予以研究因素进行处理，产生阴性结果。包括：①空白对照，不施加任何处理的对照，在动物实验中通常用以评定测量方法的准确度以及观察实验是否处于正常状态。②假处理对照，将药物用等量的药物溶剂替代，其他操作同实验组，与该组对照可帮助判断实验操作、实验环境等对实验结果的影响。

（2）阳性对照　用已知的有确切疗效的典型药物作为对照，产生阳性结果，验证实验结果的有效性。阳性对照组的结果应为阳性，若未得到设定结果，需查找实验体系、过程中可能存在的问题，此次实验结果判定无效。阳性对照包括以下几种：①标准品对照，采用标准药物或典型药物作为对照，应产生阳性结果，与实验体系中的实验药物做比较，可对比评价实验药物效价。②弱阳性对照，某些情况下，无合适的阳性对照药物或为了与实验药物作用机制相对比，采用一些疗效明确但药效不太强的药物作为对照。

（3）自身对照　同一个体接受处理前后进行对照，或对称部位进行不同处理后进行对照。处理过程中需控制其他因素相同，且观察指标较稳定。

（4）历史对照　同一实验室相同实验与以往数据对照，此对照可用于实验室质量控制。

二、药理学实验设计的要点

在开展药物的药理学实验研究前，首先需要进行实验设计，除了将上述三个基本原则运用其中，还要注意以下要点。

1.明确实验目的

根据所要解决的问题，进行实验设计，做到有的放矢，不要掺入无关的项目。

2.了解研究现状

查阅文献，了解与实验相关的实验背景、研究方法等研究现状，为自己开展研究提供一定思路和借鉴。

3.确定实验方法及观察指标

根据自己的实验设计，选择合适的动物实验模型或体外实验模型，确定分组情况，注意符合随机、对照、重复原则；根据具体的实验方法，确定实验观察指标，确保指标客观、可靠、全面。

4.给药剂量确定

（1）给药剂量换算　不同动物之间的剂量换算按照体表面积进行等量换算，并非按照体重进行换算。

（2）用药剂量的选择　实验过程中所选剂量应在该药安全剂量范围内，其药理实验才有意义。同时设定3个或以上剂量组，观察药物量效关系。进行新药研究时，剂量可参考动物实验的LD_{50}，取其1/5或1/10进行，或治疗指数在3以上的药效才有实际意义。在探索药效的最适剂量时，应从小动物开始，在整体动物实验中以2倍或3.16（$\sqrt{10}$）倍递增，在离体实验中以3倍或10倍递增。

5.给药途径、药物剂型确定

尽可能根据药物的性质采取方便的给药途径。进行新药研究时，最少要有两种给药途径：一种为口服；另一种为腹腔注射或静脉给药。

药物的剂型受药物的溶解性的影响，如水溶性的药物可以制成水溶液供口服或注射给药；油溶性的药物可制成乳状液供口服、肌内、腹腔注射；水油都难溶的药物制备成混悬液供口服给药。

6.拟定实验记录格式

实验记录一般包括以下一些内容。

（1）实验名称。

（2）实验参与者。

（3）实验样本　动物实验一般记录动物种类、品系、体重、性别；细胞实验一般记录细胞名称、获得途径等。

（4）实验药物　包括药物名称、来源、批号、纯度、剂型、配制方法等；若为自制粗提物，应有一定的质控标准，保证每次实验用药物成分含量相当。

（5）实验环境　包括时间、室温、湿度等。

（6）实验方法、步骤。

（7）实验结果记录内容及格式　可提前设计好原始记录表格，有利于实验后数据处理。

（8）实验数据处理方法　根据采集的数据不同，采取相应的数据统计处理分析方法，确保得出正确结论。

第二篇
基础药理学自主实验设计典型案例

Chapter 2

Typical Cases of Independent Experimental
Design in Basic Pharmacology

Experiment 1　Measurement of LD_{50} of Procaine Hydrochloride

Knowledge

1. The meaning, significance and measurement method of LD_{50}.
2. Mouse grouping and numbering.
3. Common calculation methods of LD_{50}.

Skill

Measure the LD_{50} and design related experiments.

Objective

Understand the drug toxicity test, and the method of measuring the median lethal dose (LD_{50}) of a certain drug.

Any new drug should undergo systematic pre-clinical researches before clinical trials, including the toxicology study to clarify the relationship between its dosage and toxic reactions, the target organ of toxic effects, and the symptom and duration of toxic reactions. Toxicology studies include acute, chronic and subacute toxicity tests. The research content, indicators, methods and requirements of any new drug preclinical toxicology research should be determined according to the drug's category.However, in principle, each study should include acute and chronic (or subacute) studies, and comply with the international GLP.

Acute toxicity test refers to the study on obvious toxic reaction of animals within 1 to 2 days after single or several administrations, which is often considered as the first step of a toxicology study. Acute toxicity tests focus on observing the toxic symptom or abnormal manifestations, and also calculate the median lethal dose (LD_{50}) and the toxic blood concentration (TC_{50}), in order to evaluate the toxicity of drugs and body's tolerance. In acute toxicity tests, when the oral dosage of chemical drugs exceeds 5 g/kg, or 100 times of common dosage for Chinese medicines, or 2 g/kg for injection dosages, but there's still no death or poisoning case, you don't have to keep increasing the dose but truthfully describe the experiment as a limit test.

Chronic toxicity test refers to observing the toxic effects of drugs on tissue structures, status of function, and metabolism, and accurately identifying the cause of death and if the toxicity is recoverable, etc., based on multiple consecutive administrations for usually 3 to 6 months. We also perform carcinogenic, teratogenic, and mutagenic tests on most drugs.

LD_{50} refers to the dose of a certain drug that can kill half of the studied animals. It is based on if the animal survives the experiment. There can be a symmetrical S-shaped curve between the logarithmic dosage and the frequency of positive cumulative death. To a certain extent, the LD_{50} reflects the acute toxicity of a drug.

There are many methods for determining the LD_{50}, but basically figure it out with statistical methods by dividing lab animals into several groups and giving different dosages of drugs to cause mortality. Calculation methods and their characteristics are listed as follows: the improved Karber's method (the Karber-Sun method), which is easy to calculate and able to provide accurate results and other related parameters. As for the sequential method, it is only suitable for drugs with rapid toxicity and has a very simple experiment process and require fewer animals, however it cannot be applied in calculating other relevant data.The weighted probability unit method (Bliss method) requires computer process, based on the linear relationship between the logarithmic dosage and probability unit. It has very accurate and reliable result, and has no special requirement for dosage in the experiment design. The count of animals in each group can also be different. It only requires that half of the groups have a response rate of more than 50%, and that of the other half should be below 50%.

Materials

1. Animals: several mice, weighing from 18 to 22 g, half male and half female.

2. Drugs: procaine hydrochloride solution.

3. Other materials: rat scale, 1 ml syringe, gastric applicator, picric acid, etc.

Methods

1. Preliminary Experiment

Initially find out the minimum dose a (0% mortality rate) and the maximum dose b (100% mortality rate), and figure out the common ratio.

（1）Determine the minimum dose a and maximum dose b of the drug

Dilute the procaine solution to one tenth, then find the 4/4 and 0/4 lethal dosage by inject 0.2 ml/10g of this drug on 8 mice.

Based on the 4/4 lethal dose, sequentially reduce the dose by 30% and test each dose on 4 mice until the death count of mice was less than 4/4. If the mortality rate of a certain dose group is 4/4, and the mortality rate is 2/4 or 3/4 after the dose is reduced by 30%, then set this dosage as b. If the mortality rate drops to 0/4 or 1/4, then set its 1.4 times as b.

Based on the 0/4 lethal dose, sequentially increase the dose by 40% and test each dose on 4 mice until the death count of mice was less than 0/4. If the mortality rate of a certain dose group is 0/4, and the mortality rate is 1/4 or 2/4 after the dose is reduced by 40%, then set this dosage as a. If the mortality rate rises to 3/4 or 4/4, then set its 1/1.4 times as a.

This method can basically ensure the mortality rate of the highest dose group is not less than 70%, and that in the lowest dosage group is not higher than 30%, in the experiment.

（2）Determine the Common Dose Ratio of Each Group, and Calculate the Dosage

Use the following formula to figure out the common ratio r (the r should be less than 1.40, generally between 1.20 and 1.26).

$$r = \sqrt[(n-1)]{b/a} \text{ (n is the count of animals)}$$

According to the common ratio r, calculate the dosage of each group as a, ar, ar^2, ar^3……ar^{n-1}, assuming the count of groups is n.

（3）Solution Preparation

Generally, we formulate drugs with the low-ratio dilution method, as different dose groups should be given same volume of drugs.

For example, if the highest dose b is 200 mg/kg, the administration volume is 0.2 ml/10 g, the common ratio r is 1.2, the count of groups is n=6, each group has 10 animals, and each animal weighs 18 to 22 g.

Firstly, find the drug concentration of the highest dose group:

$$C_1 = \frac{200 \text{ mg/kg}}{0.2 \text{ ml/10 g}} = 1\%$$

The administration volume for each group is: $V = 22 \text{ g} \times 10 \times 0.2 \text{ ml/10 g} = 4.4 \text{ ml}$ (prepare 5 ml of the solution actually)

The dispensing volume of the highest dose group:

$$V_1 = \text{The Administration Volume for Each Group} / (1-1/r) = \frac{5}{1-1/1.2} = 30 \text{ ml}$$

Accurately formulate 30 ml of 1% procaine solution, then take out 5 ml of it. Add 5 ml of normal saline to the remaining solution, and shake well, then use it to prepare drugs for the next group, and so on until the minimum dose group.

2. The Formal Experiment: calculate the LD_{50} by the Karber-Sun method

This experiment requires dosages of groups are arranged in a proportional series, the minimum dose response rate should be 0% or close to 0%, and the maximum dose response rate should be 100% or close to 100%. But you should try avoiding repeated occurrences of 0% or 100%.

（1）Randomly divide the animals into 6 groups, 10 in each group, according to their weight.

（2）Weigh and label each mouse, then intraperitoneally inject them with 0.2 ml/10g of the solution.

（3）Observe the performance and death time of animals after the administration, record the count of animal death in each group, figure out the mortality of each group, and record them in Tab. 2.1.1. Calculate the LD_{50} with the Karber-Sun method at 95% confidence interval.

（4）After the administration, the animal will illustrate increased activities in the next 1 to 2 minutes, then fall into convulsion, followed by inhibition. Finally, the animal will die. Animals that survive this experiment will recover within 15-20 minutes and won't die again, therefore you may only observe the mortality rate within 30 minutes.

3. Result Calculation

Calculate the with the Karber-Sun method:

$$LD_{50} = lg^{-1} \left[X - i\sum P - \left(\frac{3 - P_m - P_n}{4} \right) \right] \quad (mg/kg)$$

X refers the logarithmic value of the maximum dose, $i = lgr$, $P = $ mortality of each group (shown as a decimal), $\sum P$ refers the sum of mortality in each group.

The standard error (SE) of the logarithm value of $(logLD_{50})$ can be calculated according to the following formula:

$$SE = i\sqrt{(\sum P - \sum P^2)/(n-1)}$$

The i refers lgr, P is the mortality rate of each group, n is the count of animals in each group, $\sum P$ refers the sum of mortality of each group.

The 95% confidence limit of LD_{50} is: $lg^{-1} (lg\,LD_{50} \pm 1.96SE)$

You may also figure out the LD_{50} by weighted probability unit method (the Bliss method) with some calculation softwares, then figure out the LD_5 and LD_1 according to the fitting curve, in order to find the safety range and reliable safety factor of the drug.

Results

Table 2.1.1　Acute Toxicity of Procaine Hydrochloride on Mice

No.	Dosage (D) (mg/kg)	lg$D$	Count of Animal (n)	Count of Death	Death Rate (P)	P^2
1						
2						
3						
4						
5						
6						

Notes

1. Accurately prepare the solution and administrate the drug.

2. State animal strains, species, body weight, route of administration, and observation time in the experiment report, as all of them may affect the result.

3. The operation between each group should be parallel to avoid the operation error or bias among groups.

Homework

1. How to evaluate the safety of a new drug according to the result of its acute toxicity test?
2. What is the significance of therapeutic index and safety range in clinical practice?

案例一　盐酸普鲁卡因半数致死量 LD$_{50}$ 的测定

知识要求

1. 掌握 LD$_{50}$ 的含义、测定意义、方法和步骤。
2. 熟悉小鼠的随机分组、编号。
3. 了解计算 LD$_{50}$ 的常用方法。

能力要求

学会 LD$_{50}$ 的测定方法，设计完成其他药物的测定。

【实验目的】

了解药物急性毒性试验概念，掌握药物的半数致死量（LD$_{50}$）的测定方法。

【实验原理】

任何新药在进行临床药物试验前均应进行系统的临床前药物研究，其中包括药物的毒理研究，目的在于弄清药物剂量与毒性反应的关系、毒性作用的靶器官、毒性反应的表现及时间过程。毒性研究的主要内容包括：急性毒性试验、慢性毒性试验，以及亚急性毒性试验。每一种新药临床前毒理的研究内容、观察指标、方法和技术要求根据该药的申报类别确定。但原则上都应包括急性和慢性（亚急性）研究，并应符合国际通行的 GLP 标准。

急性毒性试验是指单次或数次给药后，在1~2天内动物产生的明显毒性反应的研究，常作为毒性研究的第一步。急性毒性试验的观察重点在毒性症状或异常表现，同时计算半数致死量（LD$_{50}$）或半数中毒血浓度（TC$_{50}$），以便大致推断药物的毒性程度和机体的耐受情况。急性毒性实验中，口服途径给药量，若化学药超过5 g/kg，中药超过相当于临床人用量的100倍以上，注射剂量超过2 g/kg仍未死亡或中毒时，应如实描述实验情况，不必再提高剂量继续实验，此称为限度试验。

慢性毒性试验是指在连续多次给药（常为3~6个月）的基础上观察药物对全身器官的组织形态、功能状态、生化代谢的毒性影响，并准确鉴定致死原因、毒性反应是否可恢复等。对大多数药物还应进行致癌、致畸、致突变等实验观察。

LD_{50}是指药物能使半数动物死亡的剂量，以动物死亡与否为指标。药物的对数剂量与累积死亡的阳性频数之间呈对称"S"形曲线，引起50%动物死亡所需剂量（LD_{50}）能在一定程度上反映药物急性毒性强度。

LD_{50}测定的方法很多，基本程序都是将动物分成若干组，每组给予不同的药物剂量使其产生不同的死亡率，再用统计方法求算LD_{50}。计算方法和特点如下：①改良寇氏法（Karber氏法）计算简便，结果较准确，可计算出其他有关参数。②序贯法只适用于毒性或效应出现较快的药物，其优点是测定药物的LD_{50}实验简便，可节约动物，但不能计算其他有关数据。③加权概率单位法（Bliss氏法）采用计算机处理，原理为对数剂量与概率单位呈直线关系，其计算结果准确可靠，在实验设计时对剂量之间关系没有明显要求，各组动物数也可不同，要求约一半组数的反应率在50%以上，另一半约在50%以下。

【实验材料】

1.动物及药品　体重18~22 g小鼠，雌雄各半；盐酸普鲁卡因溶液。

2.其他材料　鼠秤、1 ml注射器、苦味酸等。

【实验方法与步骤】

1.预实验

初步摸出最小剂量a（死亡率为0）和最大剂量b（死亡率为100%），并求出公比。

（1）确定药物的最小剂量a和最大剂量b　采用10倍稀释的盐酸普鲁卡因溶液，按0.2 ml/10 g各取4只小鼠，找出4/4和0/4致死剂量。

以4/4致死剂量为基础，依次按30%递减给药量，每个剂量再各试4只小鼠，直到小鼠死亡率小于4/4。若某剂量组死亡率为4/4，剂量减少30%后死亡率为2/4或3/4，则该剂量设定为b，若死亡率降到0/4或1/4，则该剂量的1.4倍设为b。

以0/4致死剂量为基础，依次按40%递增给药量，每个剂量再各试4只小鼠，直到小鼠死亡率大于0/4。若某剂量组死亡率为0/4，剂量增加40%后死亡率为1/4或2/4，则该剂量设定为a，若死亡率升至3/4或4/4，则该剂量的1/1.4倍设定为a。

此方法基本可保证正式实验时最高剂量组死亡率不低于70%，最低剂量组死亡率不高于30%。

（2）确定各组剂量公比，计算各组给药剂量

按下式公式求出公比r（r应小于1.40，一般1.20~1.26）。

$$r = \sqrt[(n-1)]{b/a} \quad （n为正式试验中动物组数）$$

按预试验中算出的公比r，则可计算出各组的给药剂量分别为a、ar、ar^2、ar^3……ar^{n-1}，假设动物组数为n。

（3）溶液的配制　要求不同剂量组在正式实验过程中所给的药物体积数相同，一般采用低比稀释法配药。

如：最高剂量为b=200 mg/kg，给药体积为0.2 ml/10 g，公比r=1.2，组数n=6，每组

动物10只，每只动物体重18~22 g。

先求最高剂量组药物浓度：

$$C_1 = \frac{200 \text{ mg/kg}}{0.2 \text{ ml/10g}} = 1\%$$

每组需用药物体积为：$V = 22 \text{ g} \times 10$ 只 $\times 0.2$ ml/10 g = 4.4 ml（实际配5 ml）

最高剂量组配药体积 $V_1 =$ 每组药液量 /（1−1/r）= $\dfrac{5}{1-1/1.2}$ = 30 ml

首先用原液精确配制 30 ml 1% 的普鲁卡因溶液，取出 5 ml 作为实验注射用药，剩余的溶液加入 5 ml 生理盐水，混匀，作为下一个剂量浓度，依次类推，每次配好的溶液取 5 ml 作为注射用药，剩余的补加 5 ml 生理盐水就稀释为下一个剂量的药物，直到配至最小剂量为止。

2. 正式试验（改良寇氏法计算 LD_{50}，由中国药学家孙瑞元改进，称寇-孙法）

本实验要求各组间剂量按等比级数排列，并要求最小剂量的反应率为 0，最大剂量反应率为 100% 或接近 0 或 100%，（但尽量避免重复出现 0% 或 100%）。

（1）根据动物的体重，随机分为 6 组，每组 10 只。

（2）按 0.2 ml/10 g 给各只小鼠逐只称重、标记、腹腔注射给药。

（3）观察给药后动物表现、死亡时间，记录各组动物死亡数，分别算出各组死亡率，并记录于表 2-1-1，寇氏法求 LD_{50} 及其 95% 可信区间。

（4）动物给药后，约 1~2 分钟表现为自主活动增加，继而惊厥，然后转入抑制，最后死亡，不死亡的动物在 15~20 分钟内恢复正常，不会再死亡，因此本实验观察 30 分钟内的死亡率即可结束实验。

3. 结果计算

用改良寇氏公式简便计算 LD_{50}：

$$LD_{50} = \lg^{-1}\left[X-i\sum P-\left(\frac{3-P_m-P_n}{4}\right)\right] \quad (\text{mg/kg})$$

式中，X 表示 最大剂量对数值；$i = \lg r$；P 表示各组动物死亡率（用小数表示）；$\sum P$ 表示各组动物死亡率总和。

LD_{50} 的对数值（$\log LD_{50}$）的标准误 SE 可按下面公式计算：

$$SE = i\sqrt{\left(\sum P - \sum P^2\right)/(n-1)}$$

式中，i 表示 $\lg r$；P 表示各组动物的死亡率；n 为各剂量组所用动物数；$\sum P$ 表示各组动物死亡率总和。

LD_{50} 的 95% 可信限为：$\lg^{-1}(\lg LD_{50} \pm 1.96 SE)$

如果有相应的计算软件，可用加权概率单位法（Bliss）法计算 LD_{50} 值，并根据拟合曲线，求出 LD_5，LD_1 的数值，以便于求药物的安全范围及可靠安全系数。

【实验结果】

表 2-1-1　盐酸普鲁卡因对小鼠的急性毒性作用

组别	剂量D （mg/kg）	lgD	动物数n（只）	死亡数（只）	死亡率P	P^2
1						
2						
3						
4						
5						
6						

【注意事项】

1.本实验定量测定药物的效价，配制溶液浓度及给药量必须准确。

2.动物的品系、种类、体重、给药途径及观察时间均会影响的结果，因此在实验报告中应注明。

3.本实验若为全班同学共同完成，尽量每个剂量组之间的操作是平行的，即应消除各组之间人为操作误差。

【思考题】

1.如何根据新药的急性毒性实验结果评价药物的安全性？

2.治疗指数和安全范围有什么实际意义？

Experiment 2　Observing the Analgesic Effect of Drugs by Writing and Hot Plate Methods

Analgesics relieve pain, and can be classified into strong and weak analgesics according to the strength of their effects. Strong analgesics refer to those that can inhibit the central pain area, including addictive analgesics, also known as narcotics, such as opioids. Whereas weak analgesics, or antipyretic analgesics, such as aspirin, means analgesics that act on peripheral pain receptors.

Nerve fibres transmit various injury signals to the spinal cord, and finally reach the sensory area of the cerebral cortex to cause pain. However, analgesics can achieve effects by inhibiting the sensory centre or reducing pain afferents. Central analgesics are easy to prove in animal experiments, while the effects of peripheral analgesics are difficult to determine.

We commonly apply physical (thermal, electrical, mechanical) and chemical pain-causing methods to screen analgesics according to the experiment purpose. Physical stimulations are suitable for screening narcotic analgesics, and chemical stimulations are suitable for screening antipyretic analgesics.

Experiment 2.1 Observe the Analgesic Effect of Drugs by Chemical Stimulations

Knowledge

1. The method of replicating pain models by chemical stimulation.
2. Methods of judging analgesic effects.
3. The mechanism of analgesics.

Skill

1. Replicate acetic-acid-induced pain model.
2. Judge and evaluate the analgesic effect.
3. Screen analgesics by pharmacology experiments.

Objective

Observe the analgesic effects of drugs, screen analgesics by chemical stimulations, and compare the analgesic effect among drugs.

Background

Sensory nerves widely distribute in the peritoneum, therefore we can replicate pain models by injecting chemical stimuli, such as acetic acid, into mice's abdominal cavity. Mouse in pain illustrates a writhing response, including a bilateral depression in the abdomen, twisted body, extended hind limbs, and raised hip. Anodynes, such as morphine, have analgesic effects to significantly inhibit this response.

Materials

1. Animals: 3 mice, weighing from 18 to 22 g, male or female

2. Drugs: 0.1% morphine hydrochloride, 4% aspirin, 0.6% acetic acid, normal saline, picric acid.

2. Other materials: rat scale, 1 ml syringe, gavage tube, etc.

Methods

1. Weigh and mark 3 mice, then observe their normal activities.

2. Administrate 0.15 ml/10g of 0.1% morphine hydrochloride intraperitoneally, 4% aspirin by gavage, and normal saline by gavage, respectively, in mice in each group.

3. 30 minutes after the administration, intraperitoneally inject each mouse with 0.3 ml of 0.6% acetic acid solution. Observe and record whether the writhing reaction occurs within 10 minutes. Record its occur times as well.

4. Record the result in Table 2.2.1, then calculate the increased percentage of pain threshold based on results from the whole class, then analyse and summarise the study result.

$$\text{The Increased Percentage of Pain Threshold (\%)} = \frac{N_2(\text{Experiment Group}) - N_2(\text{Control Group})}{N_1(\text{Control Group})} \times 100\%$$

Table 2.2.1　Effects of Drugs on Chemical Stimulation–Induced Pain in Mice

Drug	Count of Animals	Count of Animals with Writhing Reaction(N_1)	Average Count of Writhing Reactions Times	Count of Animals without Writhing Reaction(N_2)	The Increased Percentage of Pain Threshold (%)
Morphine– Hydrochloride					
Aspirin					
Normal Saline					

Notes

1. The acetic acid solution should be prepared just before the experiment.

2. Room temperature of the lab should be not lower than 10℃, otherwise the writhing reaction may occur less frequently.

3. Any one of the writhing response can be considered asa positive result. However, only when the writhing response is reduced by more than 50% can we determine its analgesic effect.

Homework

Describe the analgesic effect of morphine and aspirin and their clinical uses based on the experiment result.

Experiment 2.2 Observe the Analgesic Effect of Drugs by the Hot Plate Method

~~~~~~

Knowledge

1. Replication of pain models by the hot plate method.
2. Methods of judging analgesic effects.
3. The mechanism of analgesics.

Skill

1. Replicate pain model with the hot plate method.
2. Judge and evaluate the analgesic effect.
3. Screen analgesics by pharmacology experiments.

~~~~~~

Objective

Observe the analgesic effects of drugs, and screen analgesics by the hot plate method.

Background

Thermal stimulation acts on the body, causing the stimulated tissue producing pain-causing substances. Afterwards, this signal will reach the sensory area of the cerebral cortex to cause pain. We may place mice on a hot constant-temperature metal plate of 55 ± 0.5°C to induce pain models. After being stimulated, mice may lick and kick their hind legs, or jumping. However, analgesics can increase the pain threshold, extending the duration before the occurrence of pain response or the degree of pain.

Materials

1. Animals: mice, weighing from 18 to 22 g, female.

2. Drugs: 0.1% morphine hydrochloride, 4% aspirin, and normal saline.

3. Other materials: woolfe hot plate (constant-temperature water bath, thermometer, controller, copper plate, etc.), rat scale, 1 ml syringe, gavage tube, picric acid, etc.

Methods

1. Prepare the Hot Plate

Adjust and keep the water temperature at $(55\pm0.5)°C$.

2. Determine the Normal Pain Threshold of Mice, and Select and Group Them

Put the mouse on the hot plate, then start to record the time. Closely observe the mouse's reactions, considering licking hind foot as a signal of pain. When find this response, immediately turn off the stopwatch and record the time. This duration represents the thermal pain threshold of the mouse. Afterwards, remove the mouse to avoid scalding its foot. Discard those mice who show no response in more than 30 seconds. Choose 9 mice that illustrate pain reactions in 30 seconds, then weigh and number them into 3 groups. Measure their thermal pain threshold twice (with an interval of 3 min), and take the average value as the pre-administration pain threshold.

3. Administration and Determination of Post-Administration Pain Threshold

Inject 0.15 ml/10g of 0.1% morphine intraperitoneally, 4% aspirin by gavage, and normal saline by gavage, respectively, in mice in each group. Measure mice's pain threshold at 15, 30, 45 and 60 minutes, respectively, after the administration for two times and take their average value. If the mouse shows no response in 60 seconds, remove it to avoid burning its feet. Measure the pain threshold in 60 seconds each time.

4. Record the result

Record the results in Tab. 2.2.2, then calculate the increased percentage of pain threshold based on results from the whole class. Afterwards, analyse and summarise the study result.

$$\text{The Increased Percentage of Pain Threshold (\%)} = \frac{PT_2 - PT_1}{PT_1} \times 100\%$$

PT_1: average pre-administration pain threshold; PT_2: average post-administration pain threshold

Table 2.2.2　Effects of Drugs on Hot Plate–Induced Pain in Mice

Drugs	Count of Animals	Average Pre–Administration Pain Threshold (s)	Average Post–Administration Pain Threshold (s) / The Increased Percentage of Pain Threshold (%)				
			15min	30min	45min	60min	
Morphine–Hydrochloride							
Aspirin							
Normal Saline							

Notes

1. If possible, use only female mice in this experiment, as the scrotum of male mice may affect the result.

2. It's better to keep the room temperature at 15 to 20℃ , or the mouse may act slowly, or become very sensitive and jump easily. Avoid changing lab environment during the experiment, including light and sound.

3. If the average post-administration pain threshold is smaller than the average pre-administration pain threshold, count its result as 0.

4. Without Woolfe hot plate, you can put a 1000ml beaker in the constant temperature water bath, keep the bottom of it touching the water surface as a replacement.

Homework

Compare the characteristic of different pain models, which drugs can be applied in studying their analgesic effects respectively?

案例二　扭体法和热板法观察药物的镇痛作用

镇痛药能缓解疼痛，根据作用强弱可分为强镇痛药和弱镇痛药，强镇痛药指抑制中枢痛觉区的镇痛药，包括成瘾性镇痛药又称麻醉性镇痛药（如阿片类镇痛药）；弱镇痛药指作用于外周痛觉感受器的镇痛药，称为解热镇痛药（如阿司匹林）。

伤害引起的疼痛性刺激通过感觉纤维传入脊髓，最后到达大脑皮层感觉区引起疼痛。镇痛药可通过感觉中枢整合作用以及抑制或减少痛觉传入达到镇痛作用。中枢性镇痛药在动物实验中较易证实，而外周性镇痛药的镇痛作用不易测定。

筛选镇痛药常用的致痛方法有物理性（热、电、机械）和化学性刺激法。由于致痛原因各异，其适用场合也不同。机械刺激法、电刺激法、热刺激法适用于筛选麻醉性镇痛药，化学刺激法适用于筛选解热镇痛药。

实验一　化学刺激法观察药物的镇痛作用

知识要求
1.掌握化学刺激法疼痛模型的复制原理、方法，镇痛作用的判定方法。
2.熟悉镇痛药的作用机制。

能力要求
1.掌握醋酸疼痛模型复制及药物镇痛作用判定。
2.掌握镇痛药的筛选方法。

【实验目的】
　　观察药物的镇痛作用；学习用化学刺激法筛选镇痛药，并比较药物镇痛效果。

【实验原理】
　　腹膜的感觉神经分布广泛，将醋酸等化学刺激物注入腹腔，使小鼠产生疼痛反应，其表现为腹部双侧凹陷，躯体扭曲，后肢伸展，臀部高起，称扭体反应。吗啡等药物有镇痛作用，可明显抑制扭体反应。

【实验材料】
　　1. **动物及药品**　小鼠3只，体重18~22 g，雌雄不限；0.1%盐酸吗啡溶液，4%阿司匹林，0.6%醋酸溶液，生理盐水，苦味酸等。
　　2. **其他材料**　鼠秤、1 ml注射器、灌胃针等。

【实验方法与步骤】
　　1. **称重**　取小鼠3只，称重、标记，观察正常活动。
　　2. **给药**　各组小鼠分别腹腔注射0.1%盐酸吗啡溶液、灌胃给以4%阿司匹林溶液、生理盐水，给药体积为0.15 ml/10 g。
　　3. **观察指标**　给药30分钟后，各动物均腹腔注射0.6%醋酸溶液0.3 ml/只，观察记录小鼠注射醋酸后10分钟内是否出现扭体反应，并记录扭体次数。
　　4. **结果处理**　实验结果记录于表2-2-1。汇总全班实验结果，并计算药物痛阈提高百分率，分析结果并得出结论。

$$痛阈提高百分率（\%）=\frac{给药组无扭体反应动物数-对照组无扭体反应动物数}{对照组扭体反应动物数}\times100\%$$

表 2-2-1　药物对小鼠化学刺激法所致疼痛的影响

药物	动物数(只)	扭体反应动物数(只)	平均扭体反应次数(次)	无扭体动物数	痛阈提高百分率(%)
盐酸吗啡					
阿司匹林					
生理盐水					

【注意事项】

1.醋酸溶液应新鲜配制。

2.室温不宜低于10℃，否则扭体反应出现率低。

3.扭体反应有任何一项表现即可判定为阳性，扭体反应次数减少50%以上，才能认为有镇痛效力。

【思考题】

结合实验结果，说明吗啡、阿司匹林的镇痛效果与临床用途。

实验二　热板法观察药物的镇痛作用

知识要求

1.掌握热板法疼痛模型的复制原理、方法，镇痛作用判定方法。

2.熟悉镇痛药的作用机制。

能力要求

1.熟练掌握热板法疼痛模型复制及镇痛效果判定。

2.掌握镇痛药的筛选方法。

【实验目的】

观察药物对热刺激所致疼痛作用；了解热板法筛选镇痛药的方法。

【实验原理】

热刺激作用于机体局部，可使被刺激组织产生致痛物质，通过感觉纤维传入脊髓，最后到达大脑皮层感觉区引起疼痛。小鼠放置于（55±0.5）℃恒温的热金属板上，受热刺激可出现舔后足、踢后腿或跳跃疼痛反应。给予镇痛药可提高痛阈，推迟小鼠疼痛反应出现时间或疼痛程度。

【实验材料】

1.**动物及药品**　小鼠若干，体重18~22 g，雌性；0.1%盐酸吗啡溶液，4%阿司匹林溶液，生理盐水，苦味酸等。

2.**其他材料**　Woolfe热板（恒温水浴、控制仪、温度计、铜板等），鼠秤、1ml注射器。

【实验方法与步骤】

1.**准备热板**　调节水温并保持在（55±0.5）℃。

2.**测定正常痛阈值，挑选小鼠并分组**　将小鼠放入恒温水浴的热板上，立即打开秒表计时，密切注意观察小鼠动作，以舔后足作为疼痛反应指标。当出现此动作时，立即关上秒表，记录时间。此段时间为该小鼠的热痛阈值。然后立即取出小鼠，以免烫伤小鼠足垫。如30秒以上无反应者应弃之不用。挑选反应在30秒以内的小鼠9只，称重标号，分为三组。测定各鼠热痛阈反应时间，共2次（间隔3分钟），取平均值，此值作为给药前痛阈值。

3.**给药及测定给药后痛阈值**　3组小鼠分别腹腔注射0.1%盐酸吗啡溶液、4%阿司匹林溶液、生理盐水，给药体积为0.15 ml/10 g。给药后15、30、45、60分钟各检测痛阈值2次，取其平均值。如果60秒仍无反应，立即将小鼠取出，以免时间太长烫伤足底，痛阈值计为60秒。

4.**实验结果记录于表2-2-2**　汇总全班实验结果，并计算药物痛阈提高百分率，以时间为横坐标，痛阈提高百分率为纵坐标，作图比较药物的镇痛作用。

$$痛阈提高百分率（\%）= \frac{给药后的痛阈平均值-给药前的痛阈平均值}{给药前痛阈平均值} \times 100\%$$

表2-2-2　药物对小鼠热板法所致疼痛的影响

药物	动物数（只）	给药前痛阈平均值（秒）	给药后痛阈平均值（秒）/痛阈提高百分率（%）			
			15分钟	30分钟	45分钟	60分钟
盐酸吗啡						
阿司匹林						
生理盐水						

【注意事项】

1.小鼠宜选择雌性，因雄性鼠遇热阴囊松弛与热板接触而影响实验。

2.室温恒定在15~20℃左右较好，温度过低小鼠反应迟钝，过高则敏感，易产生跳跃动作而影响实验；避免实验周围环境的改变，如光线、声音等。

3.如给药后平均痛阈-给药前平均痛阈为负数则以0计算。

4.若无woolfe热板，亦可将1000 ml烧杯放入恒温水浴内，使烧杯底部触及水面。调节水温，使之恒定在（55±0.5）℃。

【思考题】

比较不同的疼痛模型的特点，判断哪些药物可用于镇痛效果的研究？

Experiment 3　Anticoagulant Effect of Drugs

Knowledge

1. The slide method for evaluating anticoagulant drugs.
2. The method of animal blood sampling.
3. The mechanism of anticoagulant effect of drugs.
4. Other methods of coagulation determination.

Skill

1. Blood sampling from the tip of the mouse tail.
2. Determine the end point of coagulation with the slide method.
3. Understand the process of blood coagulation and its mechanism.
4. Accurately explain the phenomena in this experiment.

Objective

Learn measuring the clotting time by the slide method, observe the anticoagulant effect of drugs, and analyse its mechanism.

Background

Normally, blood remains fluid in the circulatory system, based on the dynamic balance between blood coagulation and anticoagulation. Hence, some substances that affect the blood coagulation or fibrinolysis process can be applied as coagulation or anticoagulant drugs. Anticoagulant drugs are important substances to prevent or treat thrombosis, and it is necessary to study their mechanism.

Preliminary screening of anticoagulant drugs can be carried out in vitro by observing the effect of drugs on blood coagulation and fibrinolysis time. This process is easy to operate and require no special equipment. Meanwhile, in animal experiments, we can induce bleeding models to analyse the effect of anticoagulants, such as administrating mice with dicoumarin to form hypocoagulation.

Clotting time refers to the time required for isolated blood to clot. Any substances that can affect the activity or quantity of coagulation factors can influence the coagulation process. By measuring the clotting time, we can evaluate the anticoagulant effect of the tested drug.

Materials

1. Animals: several mice, weighing from 18 to 22 g, male or female.

2. Drugs: 0.06% aspirin suspension and 0.05% ozagrelum solution.

3. Other materials: rat scale, 1 ml syringe, picric acid, glass slide, scalpels, and clean needle, etc.

Methods

1. Grouping and Administration

Weigh and label the mice into 2 groups. Afterwards, administrate them with 0.2 ml/10 g of normal saline or aspirin suspension by gavage, respectively, once a day for 4 consecutive days. Besides, intraperitoneally inject mice in other 2 groups with normal saline or 0.2 ml/10g of 0.05% ozagrelum, respectively, once a day for 4 consecutive days.

2. Blood Sampling

Cut off the tip of the mouse tail with a razor blade, then place two drops of blood on a clean glass slide with a diameter of 5 to 10mm. Immediately record the time when the blood dropped on the slide.

3. Observation

Stir the blood with a dry needle every 30 seconds. Record the time when find the blood ropy as the clotting time. Use the other drop of blood as a parallel sample.

4. Record the result

Record data in Tab. 2.3.1 and manage data from the whole class, then figure out the increased percentage of prolongation of clotting time. Afterwards, analyse the study result, summarise the conclusion.

Increased Percentage of Prolongation of Clotting Time（%）

$$= \frac{\text{Clotting Time of the Tested Drug-Clotting Time of the Control Group}}{\text{Clotting Time of the Control Group}} \times 100\%$$

Results

Table 2.3.1　The effect of Drugs on the Clotting Time of Mice Determined by the Slide Method

Group	Dosage（mg/kg）	Count of Animals	Clotting Time（s）	Increased Percentage of Prolongation of Clotting Time
Control Group 1				
Aspirin				
Control Group 2				
Ozagrelum				

Notes

1. It's better to keep the room temperature at 14 to 18℃ during the experiment.

2. In fact, stir blood drops will affect the clotting time, so the accuracy of this study is not perfect. Therefore, this method is only suitable for preliminary screening drugs.

3. All equipments in this experiment, especially the slide and needles, must be cleaned and dried.

4. The clotting time of normal mice is 0.5 to 2 minutes.If the blood hasn't coagulated in 10 minutes, then record its clotting time as 10 minutes.

Homework

1. Are there any other methods to measure the clotting time?

2. What is the anticoagulant mechanism of ozagrelum and aspirin, and what are their characteristics?

案例三　药物的抗凝血作用

知识要求

1.掌握玻片法测定抗凝血药物的要点；动物的采血方法。

2.熟悉抗凝血药的作用机制。

3.了解其他凝血测定方法。

能力要求

1.掌握小鼠尾尖采血方法；玻片法测定凝血时间。

2.理解血液凝固过程和药物作用原理，合理解释实验现象。

【实验目的】

学习玻片法测定凝血时间的方法；观察药物的抗凝血作用，分析药物作用机制。

【实验原理】

正常情况下，血液在血循环系统中保持流体状态，这依赖于血液的凝血与抗凝过程保持动态平衡。一些影响血凝过程或纤维蛋白溶解作用的物质可以作为促凝或抗凝药物。抗凝药物是预防和治疗血栓形成的重要物质，寻找新的抗凝药物以及深入研究抗凝作用环节和机制是十分必要的。

研究药物抗凝作用初筛实验可在体外试管内进行，观察药物对血凝及纤维蛋白溶解时间的影响，操作简单，无须特殊设备；动物实验可制备出血病理模型，如小鼠服用双香豆素形成低凝血症，用抗凝药治疗，分析药物作用。

凝血时间是指血液从离体到凝固所需的时间。凡是影响凝血因子活性或数量的因素都可以影响机体的凝血过程。测定凝血时间可以观察受试药物对血凝快慢的影响。

【实验材料】

1.**动物及药品** 小鼠若干只，体重18~22 g，雌雄不限；0.06%阿司匹林混悬液，0.05%奥扎格雷溶液，生理盐水，苦味酸等。

2.**其他材料** 鼠秤、1 ml注射器、载玻片、手术刀、清洁的针头等。

【实验方法与步骤】

1.**分组、给药** 小鼠称重、标记、分组。两组小鼠分别按0.2 ml/10 g灌胃给以生理盐水、阿司匹林混悬液，连续灌胃4天，每天1次。另外两组小鼠分别腹腔注射等量生理盐水、0.05%奥扎格雷溶液0.2 ml/10 g，连续4天，每天1次。

2.**取血** 实验当日取小鼠，用刀片割尾尖，滴两滴血于干净的载玻片上，直径5~10 mm，血滴于载玻片立即计时。

3.**观察指标** 隔30秒，用干燥的针头在其中一滴血中挑动一次，至能挑起血丝为止，此为凝血时间，另一滴血作为平行测定。

4.**结果处理** 实验结果记录于表2-3-1。对全班实验结果进行统计，计算凝血时间延长百分率，分析实验结果并得出结论。

$$凝血时间延长百分率（\%）= \frac{试验药凝血时间-对照组凝血时间}{对照组凝血时间} \times 100\%$$

【实验结果】

表2-3-1 玻片法测定药物对小鼠凝血时间的影响

组别	剂量（mg/kg）	动物数（只）	凝血时间（秒）	凝血时间延长百分率
对照组1				
阿司匹林组				
对照组2				
奥扎格雷				

【注意事项】

1.实验时环境温度控制在14~18℃为宜。

2.挑动血滴会影响凝血时间，准确性较差，该法可作为初筛测试药物的凝血效果。

3.所用器材尤其载玻片及针头需提前清洗干燥。

4.正常小鼠凝血时间在0.5~2分钟，若超过10分钟未凝固记作10分钟。

【思考题】

1.除了玻片法还有哪些测定血液凝固的方法？

2.奥扎格雷和阿司匹林抗凝血的作用原理是什么，各有什么特点？

Experiment 4   The Anti–Inflammatory Effect of Glucocorticoids

Knowledge

1. The basic pathological process of inflammation.
2. The basic method of anti-inflammatory experiments.
3.The anti-inflammatory mechanism of glucocorticoids.

Skill

1. Replicate inflammation models with carrageenan solution.
2. Judge the anti-inflammatory effect of drugs.
3. Screen anti-inflammatory drugs.

Objective

Observe the inhibitory effect of glucocorticoids on partial skin inflammation in rats. Learn common experiment methods to screen anti-inflammatory drugs, especially the double-blind experiment method to avoid the influence of subjective factors.

Background

As inflammation is a common but very complicated clinical symptom, it is quite difficult to prepare a perfect inflammation animal model.Therefore, researches on the anti-inflammatory effect of a certain drug are mainly based on the comprehensive evaluation of the drug's efficacy in various models. Indicators for evaluating this effect should be objective and easy to statistically manage, including the swelling level, capillary permeability, leukocyte migration, and granulation hyperplasia, etc.

Inflammation caused by topical application of carrageenan can cause the increase in prostaglandin synthesis and edema together with vasoactive amines and kinins.This is a common method to induce inflammatory edema, with the advantages of small individual difference, high sensitivity and good repeatability. However, it has poor specificity, and some non-anti-inflammatory drugs are also effective on this kind of edema. In order to measure the swelling, you can measure the perimeter of the animal's foot with a soft ruler, or its thickness with a micrometer, or the volume of the foot.

Glucocorticoid drugs have anti-inflammatory, anti-viral, anti-shock and anti-immune effects. In this experiment, we observe the anti-inflammatory effect of drugs by apply glucocorticoids on the carrageenan-induced swelling of rats.

Materials

1. Animals: several rats, weighing from 120 to 150 g, male or female.

2. Drugs: 0.5% prednisolone or 0.5% dexamethasone injection, normal saline, 2.5% carrageenan (weigh 25 mg of it then dissolve with 1 ml saline each time before use).

3. Other materials: rat scale, syringes (0.25 ml, 1 ml and 5 ml), gavage needle, rat cage, soft ruler, spiral micrometer.

Methods

1. Grouping

Weigh and group 4 rats, then measure the perimeter of their left ankle joints and the thickness of the plantar with a soft ruler and a spiral micrometer, respectively.

2. Administration

Intraperitoneally inject rats in the experiment group with 10 mg/kg of 0.5% dexamethasone, and equal volume of normal saline for rats in the control group. 45 minutes later, subcutaneously inject 0.1 ml of 2.5% carrageenan into the middle of each rat's left plantar to cause inflammation.

3. Measurement

Measure the perimeter of the rat's ankle joint and the thickness of its foot at 10, 20, 30, 60, and 90 min, respectively, after determining inflammation. Measure at the same position to reduce bias. Observe the degree of congestion and edema as well.

4. Record results

The swelling degree refers to the difference of the thickness or perimeter of the inflamed foot plantar and that before inflammation. Gain results from the whole class, then draw a time-response chart with the swelling degree as the ordinate, and time (in minute) as the abscissa.

Results

Table 2.4.1　Effects of Prednisolone on Carrageenan-Induced Foot Swelling in Rats

No.	Weight (g)	Dosage (mg/kg)	Thickness/ Perimeter of the Rat's Inflamed Foot (mm)	The Swelling Degree of Foot and Plantar (mm)				
				10'	20'	30'	60'	90'

Notes

1. The carrageenan solution must be prepared just one day before use and stored in a refrigerator at 4℃.

2. Measure the thickness of the rat's foot at the same position to avoid bias.

3. Rats weighing from 120 to 150 g are very sensitive to inflammatory agents, with high swelling and small individual differences.

Homework

1. What are the two categories of anti-inflammatory drugs?

2. What are the anti-inflammatory mechanism and characteristics of glucocorticoids?

案例四   糖皮质激素的抗炎作用

知识要求

1. 掌握炎症的基本病理过程；抗炎实验的基本方法。

2. 熟悉糖皮质激素类药物的药理作用及机制。

能力要求

1. 掌握角叉菜胶溶液致炎模型及抗炎作用判定方法。

2. 掌握抗炎药物筛选方法的基本要领。

【实验目的】

观察糖皮质激素对大鼠部分皮肤局部炎症反应的抑制作用；学习筛选抗炎药常用的实验方法（采用双盲法实验，可避免主观因素的影响）。

【实验原理】

炎症是常见的临床症状，其过程是一个相当复杂的病理生理过程，要制备完善的动物模型是相当困难的。因此，对某个药物的抗炎作用研究，主要依据该药物在多种炎症模型中的治疗功效来综合评价、分析。炎症指标的选择应该客观并易于统计处理，主要有肿胀度、毛细血管通透性、白细胞游走、肉芽增生等。

局部应用角叉菜胶引起炎症，前列腺素合成明显增加，并与血管活性胺类和激肽类物质一起诱发水肿。本法是较为广泛应用的炎症性水肿模型，具有差异性小，敏感性高、重复性好等优点。但本法特异性低，一些非抗炎药同样有效。肿胀的测定方法可以用软尺测量足跖周长，也可用千分尺测定足跖厚度或测定足跖体积。

糖皮质激素类药物具有抗炎、抗病毒、抗休克及抗免疫等作用，本实验通过致炎物引起大鼠足跖炎症性肿胀，观察药物的抗炎症渗出作用。

【实验材料】

1. 动物及药品　大鼠120~150g左右，性别不限；0.5%泼尼松龙注射液或0.5%地塞米松注射液，生理盐水，2.5%角叉菜胶溶液。

2. 其他材料　鼠秤，1 ml注射器，0.25 ml注射器，5 ml注射器，大鼠灌胃针头，鼠笼，软皮尺，螺旋测微器。

【实验方法与步骤】

1. 分组　大鼠4只称重，软皮尺和螺旋测微器分别测量左踝关节周长和足跖厚度，分组。

2. 给药　给药组大鼠腹腔注射0.5%地塞米松注射液10 mg/kg，对照组大鼠注射等容积的生理盐水，45分钟后分别在各鼠左跖中部皮下注射2.5%角叉菜胶溶液0.1 ml。

3. 观察指标　致炎后10分钟、20分钟、30分钟、60分钟、90分钟测定其踝关节周长和足跖厚度，注意每次测量的部位要一致，尽可能减少误差，注意观察足跖充血水肿的程度。

4. 结果处理　所得结果以致炎后减去致炎前足跖厚度或周长为肿胀度，统计全班结果，以肿胀度为纵坐标，时间（分钟）为横坐标绘图，画出时程反应图。

【实验结果】

表 2-4-1　腹腔注射泼尼松龙对角叉菜胶致大鼠足肿胀的影响

编号	体重（g）	剂量（mg/kg）	左后足正常周长/厚度（mm）	足跖肿胀度（mm）				
				10′	20′	30′	60′	90′

【注意事项】

1. 角叉菜胶溶液须在临用前一天配制，置4 ℃冰箱保存。

2. 测定足跖厚度部位须一致，否则误差较大。

3. 体重120~150 g的大鼠对致炎剂最敏感，肿胀度高，差异性小。

【思考题】

1. 抗炎药分为哪两大类？

2. 糖皮质激素的抗炎作用特点和机制是什么？

Experiment 5　The Catharsis Effect of Magnesium Sulfate on Mice

Knowledge

1. The catharsis mechanism of magnesium sulfate.
2. The method of measuring the advancement of intestinal contents.
3. Pharmacological effects and clinical applications of magnesium sulfate.

Skill

1. Anatomy skills on mouse gastrointestinal tracts.
2. Measure the length of intestinal tubes.

Objective

Observe the effect of magnesium sulfate on intestinal tracts, and analyse its catharsis mechanism.

Background

We usually study the effect of drugs on the motility of gastrointestinal tract smooth muscles with experiments on isolated animal intestines or in vivo gastric emptying and intestinal propulsion experiments.

This simple and safe experiment provides rough data of the advancement of the contents of the intestine, using ink as the tracer. However, it can not provide details, such as the effect of drugs on the contraction of intestines. This method can also be used to study the bioelectric activities.

Magnesium and sulfate ions are both not easily absorbed to the intestinal tract. After entering the intestine, the magnesium sulfate can increase the osmotic pressure and water volume in it, promoting intestinal peristalsis and catharsis.

Materials

1. Animals: 2 mice, weighing from 18 to 22 g, male or female.
2. Drugs: inked sodium chloride solution and inked magnesium sulfate solution

3. Other materials: rat scale, 1 ml syringe, gavage needle, surgical scissor, ruler, etc.

Methods

1. Administration

Fast 2 mice for more than 6 hours, then weigh and number them. Afterwards, administrate them with inked sodium chloride and inked magnesium sulfate solutions respectively.

2. Observation

Execute the mice 40 minutes later. Afterwards, cut along the midline of its abdomen to observe bowel movements and intestinal distension. Next, separate the mouse's intestinal tract from the pylorus to the rectum with a surgical scissor. Stretch the intestinal tube, and measure the distance between the pylorus and the ink, and the full length of the intestine, then calculate their ratio. Observe their stool properties as well.

Results

Table 2.5.1　The Catharsis Effect of Magnesium Sulfate on Mice

Observation	Normal Control Group	Magnesium Sulfate Group
Distance from Ink to the Pylorus		
Intestine Length		
Ratio		
Peristalsis		
Distension		
Fecal Traits		

Notes

1. Gently separate the intestine from the pylorus under the stomach. Do not damage the intestine, or it may affect the observation.

2. The interval between drug administration and mice execution must be accurate.

3. Avoid pulling when cutting the intestines, or the measurement accuracy may be affected.

Homework

State the catharsis mechanism and clinical application of magnesium sulfate.

案例五　硫酸镁对小鼠的导泻作用

知识要求
1.掌握硫酸镁的导泻原理及肠道内容物推进的测定方法。
2.熟悉硫酸镁的药理作用及临床应用。
能力要求
熟练掌握小鼠胃肠道解剖结构及肠管长度测定方法。

【实验目的】

观察硫酸镁对肠道的作用，分析其导泻作用原理。

【实验原理】

药物对胃肠道平滑肌运动功能的影响，通常可用离体动物肠管或在体胃排空、肠推进运动的实验方法。本实验通过墨汁为示踪物追踪其在肠道内推进距离，该法简单、安全，然而仅能获得肠道对内容物的推进的粗略数据，不能了解药物对肠道收缩作用等细节，但可研究其生物电活动等。

硫酸镁进入肠道，其镁离子和硫酸根离子均不易被肠道吸收，肠内渗透压升高，肠腔内水分增加，促进肠蠕动而导泻。

【实验材料】

1.动物及药品　小鼠2只，体重18~22 g，雌雄不限；墨汁氯化钠溶液，墨汁硫酸镁溶液。

2.其他材料　鼠秤、1 ml注射器、灌胃针头、手术剪，尺子等。

【实验方法与步骤】

1.给药　取2只小鼠，禁食6小时以上，称重编号，分别灌胃墨汁氯化钠溶液和墨汁硫酸镁溶液。

2.观察指标　40分钟后处死小鼠，沿腹中线切开腹腔，观察肠蠕动及肠膨胀情况；手术剪分离小鼠幽门部至直肠段肠管，拉直肠管，测量肠管内墨汁距幽门的距离及肠管全长，计算两者比值；观察粪便性状。

【实验结果】

表 2-5-1　硫酸镁对小鼠的导泻作用

观察项目	正常组	硫酸镁组
墨汁距幽门距离		
肠管长度		
两者比值		
肠蠕动情况		
肠膨胀情况		
粪便性状		

【注意事项】

1.分离肠管从胃下面的幽门部开始，分离肠系膜时动作需轻，防止损伤肠管，影响内容物观察。

2.灌服药物和处死动物的时间间隔需准确，否则影响较大。

3.剪取肠道时避免牵拉，否则影响测量的准确度。

【思考题】

硫酸镁导泻原理及临床用途是什么？

Experiment 6　The Effect of Drugs Against Central Stimulant–Induced Seizures

Knowledge

1. Replication of convulsion models.
2. Methods of screening anticonvulsant drugs.
3. The mechanism of dimefline.
4. Other methods of replicating other seizure models.

Skill

1. Replicate and judge convulsion models.
2. Understand the mechanism of drugs and be able to explain the phenomenon in this study.

Objective

Observe the protective effect of sodium valproate on dimefline-induced convulsion.

Background

The convulsion is involuntary and uncoordinated twitches of skeletal muscles caused by the overexcitement of the central nervous system and mainly occur in children with high fever, eclampsia, tetanus, and acute poisoning.It can be controlled with central inhibitors or some peripheral muscle relaxants.Central stimulants, including brain stimulants and spinal cord stimulants, improve the activity of the central nervous system. However when administrated at a too large dosage or used too frequently, they may cause convulsion due to the excessive excitement of brain and medulla oblongata. After the excitement, it may turn into life-threatening prohibitive inhibition because of the exhaustion of brain energy.

Dimefline is a central stimulant that directly excites the respiratory centre. In case of overdose, it can cause convulsion. We may screen anticonvulsants and anti-epileptic drugs based on their protective effects on dimefline-induced convulsions. Inducing convulsions by chemical substances is easy to operate and does not require special equipment, and can also analyse the mechanism of the tested drug to a certain extent. It is also a common method of screening drugs for absence-like seizures.

Materials

1. Animals: 2 mice, weighing from 18 to 22 g, male or female.

2. Drugs: 2 % sodium valproate, 0.04% dimefline, and normal saline.

3. Other materials: rat scale, syringe, bell jar.

Methods

1. Grouping: number and weigh 2 mice.

2. Preventive administration: intraperitoneally inject 6 mg/10g (i.e 0.3 ml/10 g) of 2% sodium valproate and 0.3 ml/10g of normal saline to mice.

3. Convulsions and observation: 30 minutes later, subcutaneously inject 0.08 mg/10g of 0.04% dimefline to mice, then observe them, including the incubation time and intensity of reactions, such as spasm, fall, rigidity and death.

4. Record results: manage the result from the whole class in Table 2.6.1, and carry out a statistical analysis.

Results

Table 2.6.1　The Anticonvulsant Effect of Sodium Valproate

Drug	Weight (g)	Dosage	Reactions after Dimefline Injections
Sodium Valproate			
Normal Saline			

Notes

If necessary, you may replace the dimefline with subcutaneous injection at the dose of 1.2 mg/10 g of pentetrazol, which can cause more typical convulsive reactions.

Homework

Discuss the effect and clinical applications of each drug based on the study result.

案例六　药物对抗中枢兴奋药致惊厥的作用

知识要求

1. 掌握惊厥模型复制方法，抗惊厥药物筛选方法。

2. 熟悉二甲弗林的药理作用及机制。

3. 了解其他惊厥模型的复制方法。

能力要求

1. 熟练掌握化学品引起惊厥的模型复制及判定。

2. 理解药物的作用机制并能合理解释实验现象。

【实验目的】

观察丙戊酸钠对二甲弗林惊厥的保护作用。

【实验原理】

惊厥是中枢神经系统过度兴奋引起的骨骼肌不自主和不协调的抽搐。见于小儿高热、子痫、破伤风和急性中毒等情况，可用中枢性运动抑制药或某些外周性肌肉松弛药加以控制。中枢神经兴奋药可提高中枢神经系统功能活动，分为大脑兴奋药和脊髓兴奋药。此类药物使用剂量过大或使用过频时，由于大脑和延髓过度兴奋易产生惊厥；过度兴奋后，由于大脑能量耗竭，又易转为超限抑制，危及生命。

二甲弗林是直接兴奋呼吸中枢的中枢兴奋药，剂量过大时可引起惊厥反应。药物对二甲弗林所致惊厥的保护作用可用来初筛抗惊厥药和抗癫痫药。化学物质引起的惊厥反应操作简单，不需特殊仪器设备，可以在一定程度上进行作用原理分析。此方法可作为筛选癫痫小发作有效药物的常用方法。

【实验材料】

1. **动物及药品**　小鼠2只，体重18~22 g，雌雄不限；丙戊酸钠溶液，0.04%二甲弗林溶液，生理盐水。

2. **仪器设备及手术器械等**　鼠秤，注射器，钟罩。

【实验方法与步骤】

1. **分组**　取小鼠2只，编号，称重。

2. **预防给药**　小鼠分别腹腔注射2%丙戊酸钠6 mg/10 g（即0.3 ml/10 g）和生理盐水0.3 ml/10 g。

3.致惊厥后观察指标 30分钟后，小鼠皮下注射0.04%二甲弗林溶液0.08 mg/10 g，观察各鼠反应的快慢和强度（痉挛、跌倒、强直或死亡）。

4.结果处理 收集全班数据，将结果填于表2-6-1，进行统计学处理。

【实验结果】

表 2-6-1 丙戊酸钠的抗惊厥作用

组别	体重（g）	剂量	注射二甲弗林后的反应
丙戊酸钠			
生理盐水			

【注意事项】

若条件许可，可皮下注射戊四氮代替二甲弗林，戊四氮的惊厥反应较为典型，剂量为1.2 mg/10 g。

【思考题】

试根据结果讨论各药的作用及临床应用。

Experiment 7   Organophosphorus Poisoning and Rescue

Knowledge

1. The mechanism of organophosphate poisoning.
2. The mechanism of organophosphate rescue with atropine and pralidoxime iodide.
3. Symptoms of organophosphate poisoning.

Skill

1. Identify symptoms of organophosphate poisoning.
2. Measure cholinesterase activity.
3. Rescue organophosphate poisoning.

Objective

Observe symptoms of organophosphate poisoning and its inhibition to cholinesterase in blood. Besides, analyse the detoxification mechanism of atropine and pralidoxime based on their rescue effects.

Background

The organophosphate poisoning and rescue experiment is a systematic practice based on cholinergic neurophysiology and pharmacological knowledge. This study reveals not only M and N-like symptoms caused by acetylcholine accumulations, but also the nature of M and N effects. One of the most severe toxicity of organophosphate is the cholinesterase inhibition, as the degree of this inhibition is positively correlated with its symptoms. You may measure the activity of cholinesterase in blood according to the appendix to determine the level of poisoning.

Organophosphorus pesticides are long-lasting anti-cholinesterase substances, which can inhibit the cholinesterase activity, causing a large accumulation of acetylcholine and toxicity, leading to M-like and N-like symptoms. However, atropine is an M receptor blocker that can rapidly relieve M-like and some central nerve symptoms. Moreover, pralidoxime iodide is a cholinesterase resurrection drug that can restore cholinesterase activity and also directly combine with organophosphorus pesticides for excretion, in order to detoxify the organophosphorus.

Materials

1. Animals: 2 rabbits, weighing from 2.0 to 2.5 kg, male or female.

2. Drugs: 5% trichlorfon, 0.1% atropine sulfate,2.5% pralidoxime iodide.

3. Other materials: rabbit box, 5 ml syringe, pupil ruler, stopwatch, glass slide, alcohol cotton ball, dry cotton ball, etc.

Methods

1. Observe the Normal State

Weigh the rabbit then fix it in the box. Afterwards, observe its indicators as follows: respiratory rate and amplitude, pupil size, saliva secretion, urine and fece conditions, and muscle tension.

2. Observe Poisoning State

Intravenously administrate 80 mg/kg of 5% trichlorfon solution to the rabbit's ear vein, then observe the indicators above. In case of no poisoning symptom, add1/3 of the dosage again after 20 to 25 minutes.

3. Rescue after Poisoning

Intravenously inject 4.0 mg/kg of 0.1% atropine to one of the rabbit when it shows obvious poisoning symptoms, and 50 mg/kg of 2.5% pralidoxime iodide to the other one. Observe whether their poisoning symptoms are alleviated, and record all the significantly reduced indicators. In case of no amelioration, add1/3 of the dosage.

4. Record the Result

Record all data in Table 2.7.1.

Results

Table 2.7.1　Symptoms of Rabbits before and after the Organophosphate Poisoning

Rabbit	Breath	Pupil（mm）	Saliva Secretion	Urinary and fecal Excretion	Muscle Tremor
Before Poisoning					
After Poisoning					
Detoxification by Atropine					
Before Poisoning					
After Poisoning					
Detoxification by Pralidoxime Iodide					

Notes

1. Trichlorfon is a highly toxic substance that can be absorbed from the skin. In case of contact, immediately rinse with water. You must not use alkaline soap to clean it as trichlorfon transforms into even more toxic dichlorvos in alkaline conditions.

2. Clean the saliva and excrement before administrating drugs for easier observation.

3. Closely monitor the rabbit's physiological indicators and rescue them in time, or they may die.

4. Cut off the rabbit's eyelashes to measure the pupil.

5. Keep the rabbit's position unchanged and the light condition consistent during the experiment, as the pupil size is affected by light.

Homework

1. According to the experiment result, analyse the mechanism of organophosphorus pesticide poisoning and the detoxification mechanism of atropine and pralidoxime iodide.

2. Which indicators are suitable for screening organophosphorus antidote?

Appendix: Determination of Cholinesterase Activity in Blood by Colorimetric

Background

Cholinesterase hydrolyses acetylcholine into acetic acid and choline, therefore the amount of produced acetic acid, which can be measured with bromothymol blue, reflects the activity of cholinesterase. Drip a drop of blood on the test paper, the spot will be blue as its pH value is around 7.4. However, as the cholinesterase produces acetic acid, the blood spot will gradually turn red. According to the colour change of this spot, we can figure out the enzyme activity.

Methods

1. Prepare the Test Paper

Immerse the filter paper in the mix solution of acetylcholine and alcohol bromothymol blue. Weigh 0.23 g of acetylcholine bromide and 0.14g of bromothymol blue, then dissolve them with 20 ml of ethanol and adjust the pH of this system to about 8.0 with 0.4 mol/L NaOH solution.Cut the filter paper into strips for about 1cm × 30cm, and immerse it in the solution. Afterwards, take out and dry the filter paper, then cut it into squares for 1cm × 1cm. Next, store them in a dry brown bottle.

2. Enzyme Activity Determination

Place the test paper in the centre of a glass slide, then dip a drop of blood on it and immediately put another glass slide on it, spreading it to 0.6 to 0.8 cm diameter. Incubate the system at 36.7°C for 20 minutes, then take it out and compare its colour with the standard palette to determine the enzyme activity.

The judgment criteria are listed in the table below:

Table 2.7.2 The Correspondence between Colour and Cholinesterase Activity

Colour	Blue	Grey–Blue	Bronze–Brown	Brown	Brown–Red
Enzyme Activity	0	20	50	80	100

Note

Enzyme activity less than 60% indicates poisoning.

案例七　有机磷农药中毒与解救

知识要求

1.掌握有机磷中毒原理，阿托品和碘解磷定对有机磷中毒的解救作用机理。

2.熟悉有机磷中毒的症状。

能力要求

1.准确识别有机磷中毒的症状及掌握测定胆碱酯酶活性的方法。

2.掌握有机磷中毒的解救要领。

【实验目的】

观察有机磷药物中毒的症状及对血液中胆碱酯酶的抑制情况。根据阿托品和碘解磷定对有机磷中毒的解救效果，分析两者的解毒机制。

【实验原理】

有机磷中毒及解救实验是胆碱能神经生理、药理知识的系统实践，不仅能观察到体内乙酰胆碱的大量积聚而引起的M、N样症状，而且可以通过不同性质的解毒药物进一步认识M和N样作用，了解解毒剂性质，是较好描述胆碱神经系统效应的实验之一。有机磷中毒后体内最重要的改变是胆碱酯酶明显被抑制，酶活力抑制程度与临床表现呈正相关，可根据实验后附录测定全血胆碱酯酶活力，了解中毒情况。

有机磷农药为持久性抗胆碱酯酶药，进入体内后能抑制胆碱酯酶活性，造成乙酰胆碱大量蓄积从而产生毒性，表现为M样、N样症状。阿托品为M受体阻断药，能迅速解除M样症状及部分中枢症状；碘解磷定为胆碱酯酶激活药，可恢复胆碱酯酶活性，并可直接与游离的有机磷农药结合转变为无毒的物质从体内排出，从而解毒。

【实验材料】

1. 动物及药品 家兔2只，体重2.0~2.5 kg，雌雄不限；5%敌百虫溶液，0.1%硫酸阿托品，2.5%碘解磷定。

2. 其他材料 兔箱、5 ml注射器、测瞳尺、秒表、玻片、酒精棉球、干棉球等。

【实验方法与步骤】

1. 观察家兔正常状态 家兔称重、固定于兔箱，观察以下指标：呼吸频率与幅度、瞳孔大小、唾液分泌、大小便、肌张力及有无肌震颤。

2. 中毒症状观察 家兔耳缘静脉注射5%敌百虫溶液80 mg/kg，观察上述指标，如无中毒症状，20~25分钟后追加1/3剂量。

3. 中毒后解救 中毒症状明显时，其中一只立即静脉注射0.1%阿托品溶液4.0 mg/kg，另一只静脉注射2.5%碘解磷定50 mg/kg，观察中毒症状是否减轻，明显减轻可记录上述指标；未见减轻，追加上述剂量的1/3。

4. 结果处理 将结果记录于表2-7-1。

【实验结果】

表2-7-1 家兔有机磷中毒前、后及解毒后的症状表现

家兔	呼吸	瞳孔（mm）	唾液分泌	尿、粪排泄	肌震颤
中毒前					
中毒后					
阿托品解毒					
中毒前					
中毒后					
碘解磷定解毒					

【注意事项】

1. 敌百虫为剧毒药，可从皮肤吸收，如与手接触，应立即用清水冲洗，忌用碱性肥皂，因敌百虫在碱性条件下转变为毒性更强的敌敌畏。

2. 给药前擦干动物的唾液和粪、尿，利于实验观察。

3. 密切观察家兔生理指标变化，中毒时解救动作需迅速，否则家兔可能死亡。

4. 剪去家兔眼睫毛便于测量瞳孔。

5. 因瞳孔大小受光线影响，在实验过程中应保持家兔的位置不变，保持光线条件一致。

【思考题】

1. 根据实验结果，分析有机磷农药中毒机制及阿托品、碘解磷定解毒机制。

2. 将本法用于有机磷解毒剂筛选时，最好选用哪些指标？

附：比色法测定血液中胆碱酯酶活力

【原理】

胆碱酯酶能水解乙酰胆碱为醋酸和胆碱，醋酸生成量的多少可反映胆碱酯酶活力

高低。利用酸碱指示剂溴麝香草酚蓝可检测醋酸生成量。将血液滴于试纸上，由于血液pH值为7.4，血斑呈蓝色；之后胆碱酯酶水解乙酰胆碱产生醋酸，pH值下降，血斑逐渐变为红色。根据颜色改变，可判断酶的活力。

【方法】

1.检测试纸制备　滤纸浸入乙酰胆碱和溴麝香草酚蓝酒精溶液，制备成检测试纸。称取溴化乙酰胆碱0.23 g，溴麝香草酚蓝0.14 g，加无水乙醇20 ml溶解，加0.4 mol/L NaOH调节pH为8.0左右，将滤纸剪为1 cm×30 cm大小的条状，全部浸入溶液，取出晾干，剪成1 cm×1 cm大小的试纸片，保存于干燥的棕色瓶中。

2.酶活力测定　取试纸置于玻片中央，玻棒蘸一滴全血滴于纸片中央，立即盖上另一玻片，使血滴扩散成一圆形斑点（直径宜为0.6~0.8 cm），36.7℃保温20分钟取出，与标准色板比色，判断酶活力大小。判断标准如下：

表2-7-2　胆碱酯酶活力与标准色板对照表

标准色板颜色	蓝	灰蓝	棕褐	棕	红棕
胆碱酶活力	0	20	50	80	100

注：酶活力低于60%即为中毒。

Experiment 8　The Effect of Efferent Nervous System Drugs on Rabbit's Blood Pressure

Knowledge

1. Key points of rabbit anesthesia and surgery.

2. The method of measuring blood pressure by the biological signal system.

3. The formation of blood pressure and its influencing factors.

4. Targets of efferent nervous system drugs and their mechanism of influencing blood pressure.

Skill

1. Perform anesthesia and surgery on rabbits.

2. Measure the rabbit's arterial blood pressure.

3. Explain the performance of drugs in this experiment with pharmacology knowledge.

4. Design experiments to determine the blood pressure of animals.

Objective

Learn the acute anesthesia and blood pressure measurement on animals, and observe the effect of efferent nervous system drugs on rabbit's blood pressure. Understand the interaction between these drugs, and study their mechanism at the receptor level.

Background

The efferent nervous system drug involves a wide range of research and experimental methods, including the blood pressure test, a method to test the sensitivity of efferent nervous system drugs. Generally, we employ acute blood pressure studies on cats, dogs, rabbits and rats.

In terms of research content, we mainly focus on neurotransmitters, receptors and their effects. Animal or in vitro organ experiments are used in observing the effect of efferent nervous system drugs. We can also use blocking agents as tools to determine the type of these drugs. Furthermore, radioligand binding can be applied in analysing the binding effect and force between drugs and receptors. Moreover, we can also study the relationship between drugs and neurotransmitters. For short, there are plenty of pharmacological studies on neurologic drugs and numerous experiment designs.

The autonomic nervous system, a significant part of the efferent nervous system, contains the parasympathetic nervous system with acetylcholine as its transmitter, and the sympathetic nervous system with norepinephrine as its transmitter. These systems coordinate and fight with each other to maintain the body's balanced physiological function.Drugs mainly affect them with transmitters and receptors, such as relax or contract smooth muscles, influence blood pressure, drive gland secretion, etc. We can also indirectly and qualitatively analyse the type and function of receptors in different tissues.

There are many methods for measuring animal blood pressure, such as the rat tail artery blood pressure measurement method, a non-invasive measurement that does not damage the animal and can measure the animal for multiple times. In addition, the invasive intubation biosignal acquisition system is low cost and only requires a small number of animals. It can measure multiple drugs on a single animal sample, and even compare the change in blood pressure before and after the administration, benefiting the analysis of test drug mechanism.

Materials

1. Animals: 1 rabbit, weighing around 2 kg, male.

2. Drugs: normal saline, 500 U/ml sodium heparin, 2% sodium pentobarbital, 0.01% adrenaline, 0.01% norepinephrine, 0.05% isoproterenol, 1% phentolamine, 1% atropine, acetylcholine (0.0001%, 0.001%, 0.01%), 0.1% timolol.

3. Other materials: surgical instruments (scalpel, surgical scissor, ophthalmic scissor, hemostat, arterial clamp), arterial cannula, tee, pressure sensor, syringes (1 ml, 5 ml, and 10 ml), thread, baby scale, surgery table, operation light, PowerLab biological signal acquisition and processing system.

Methods

1. Instrument Calibration

Calibrate the instrument before the experiment and save the setting file. For specific methods, see user's manual of PowerLab 7.0.

2. Anesthesia

Weigh the rabbit and intravenously inject it with 1.5 ml/kg of 2% pentobarbital sodium at its ear vein, then fix it in the supine position on the operation table.

3. Operation

Dehair the middle of the rabbit's neck, then cut its skin. Bluntly separate its subcutaneous fascia and trachea. Cut a ' ⊥ '-shaped incision and intubate through it, then ligate it with a thick thread. Afterwards, perform blunt separations on deeper neck muscles to find the vascular nerve sheath, then separate the carotid artery and thread two threads under it. Ligate the artery's distal end, then clamp its proximal end with an arterial clip. Next, cut a V-shaped oblique opening at the end of the artery with the tip of an ophthalmic scissor.

4. Arterial Cannulation

Assemble the arterial cannula, the tee with the blood pressure transducer, and fill the device with 500U/ml heparin solution. After ensuring no air in it, intubate the artery towards the centripetal direction and fix it with the thread. Next, remove the clamp and observe whether the blood surface in the intubation pulsate.

5. Record the Blood Pressure Curve

Turn on the PowerLab system and record a section of normal blood pressure curve. Afterwards, inject the following drugs into the rabbit's ear vein. Immediately mark the administration time in the software and record the change in blood pressure and heart rate. Administrate the next drug after the rabbit's blood pressure returning stable.

6. Result Process

Analyse and compare the change in blood pressure and heart rate before and after drug administrations, and analyse the mechanism.

Table 2.8.1   Influences of Efferent Nervous System Drugs on the Blood Pressure of Anaesthetised Rabbits

No.	Drug	Dosage Before (μg/kg)	Drug Volume After (ml/kg)	Blood Pressure(mmHg)/ Heart Rate(/min)	
1. Observe the effect of epinephrine drugs on blood pressure					
（1）	0.01%Adrenaline	10	0.1		
（2）	0.01%Norepinephrine	10	0.1		
（3）	0.05%Isoproterenol	50	0.1		
2. Observe the effects of α –receptor blockers on blood pressure					
1%Phentolamine		1mg/kg	0.1		
Administrate the animal with the following drugs after 5 minutes					
（1）	0.01%Adrenaline	10	0.1		
（2）	0.01%Norepinephrine	10	0.1		
（3）	0.05%Isoproterenol	50	0.1		
3. Observe the effects of β –receptor blockers on blood pressure					
0.1%Timolol		0.1mg/kg	0.1		
Administrate the animal with the following drugs after 5 minutes					
（1）	0.01%Adrenaline	10	0.1		
（2）	0.01%Norepinephrine	10	0.1		
（3）	0.05%Isoproterenol	50	0.1		
4. Observe the effect of cholinergic drugs on blood pressure and cholinergic receptor blockers					
（1）	0.0001%Acetylcholine(Ach)	1	0.1		
（2）	1%Atropine	0.1mg/kg	0.2		
（3）	0.001%Ach	1	0.1		
（4）	0.01%Ach	10	0.1		

Notes

1. The anaesthetic must be injected slowly. In case of the rabbit's eyelid reflex disappears, or its breath or muscle relaxes, immediately stop the administration.

2. During the operation, except for cutting its neck skin, you should finish all other operations by blunt separation.

3. Before looking for the rabbit's common carotid artery, you should separate the trachea first, because the common carotid artery locates deep on both sides of it and it would be difficult to find them without separating them. Besides, bleedings from other blood vessels may occur as well.

4. Do not cut off the artery. However, the opening should not be too small, otherwise it will be difficult to intubate.

5. Before the intubation, make sure that there's no air in the device. After the cannula is inserted, keep it in line with the blood vessel to prevent falling out or being bent.

6. Protect the injection site.

7. Some drugs must be prepared just before use, such as adrenaline and acetylcholine, otherwise the study result may be affected. Carefully read the drug instruction before preparing the medicine to ensure its effectiveness.

8. Patiently wait until the rabbit's blood pressure and heart rate become basically stable, then enter the next phase of the experiment.

Homework

1.Discuss the similarity and difference among epinephrine, norepinephrine, and isoproterenol on the cardiovascular system.

2. How to verify the M-like and N-like effects of acetylcholine?

Appendix: The Effect of Efferent Nervous System Drugs on Rat's Blood Pressure

Materials

1. Animals: 1 rat, weighing around 400 g, male or female.

2. Drugs: 3% chloral hydrate, heparin sodium, and other medicines in Table 2.8.2.

3. Other materials: surgical instruments (same with the rabbit experiments), arterial cannula (the scalp needle is made of a plastic hose with a suitable diameter, protecting the artery from being pierced).

Methods

1. Anesthesia

Weighing then intraperitoneally inject the rat with 0.5 ml/100g of 1% pentobarbital sodium or 1 ml/100g of 3% chloral hydrate. Afterwards, fix it on the operation table in the supine position.

2. Separate the Common Carotid Artery

Cut open the middle of the rat's neck with a surgical scissor, then tear open the muscle layer with a hemostatic forceps to expose its trachea. Afterwards, find the vascular nerve sheath, and bluntly separate the two common carotid arteries, and pass two threads under the artery.

3. Arterial Cannulation

Ligate the artery's distal end, then clamp its proximal end with an arterial clip. Next, cut a V-shaped oblique opening at the end of the artery with the tip of an ophthalmic scissor. Afterwards, assemble the arterial cannula, the tee with the blood pressure transducer, and fill the device with 500U/ml heparin solution. After ensuring no air in it, intubate the artery towards the centripetal direction and fix it with the thread. Next, remove the clamp and observe whether the blood surface in the intubation pulsate.

4. Arterial Cannulation

Ligate the artery's proximal end, then clamp its distal end with an arterial clip. Next, cut a V-shaped oblique opening at the end of the artery with the tip of an ophthalmic scissor. Afterwards, assemble the arterial cannula, the tee with the blood pressure transducer, and fill the device with 500U/ml heparin solution. After ensuring no air in it, intubate the artery towards the centripetal direction and fix it with the thread. Next, remove the clamp and observe whether the blood surface in the intubation pulsate.

5. Record the Blood Pressure Curve

Turn on the PowerLab and record a section of normal blood pressure curve.

6. Administration

Administer drugs with normal saline through the arterial cannula, meanwhile record its blood pressure. Administrate the next drug after the rabbit's blood pressure returning stable.

7. Result Processing

same with the rabbit experiment.

Table 2.8.2   Influences of Efferent Nervous System Drugs on the Artery Blood Pressure of Anaesthetised Rats

No.	Drug	Dosage (μg/kg)	Drug Volume (ml/kg)	Blood Pressure(mmHg)/ Heart Rate(/min)	
				Before	After
1. Observe the effect of epinephrine drugs on blood pressure					
（1）	0.004%Adrenaline	40	0.1		
（2）	0.02%Norepinephrine	20	0.1		
（3）	0.02%Isoproterenol	200	0.1		
2. Observe the effects of α –receptor blockers on blood pressure					
1%Phentolamine		2mg/kg	0.1		
Administrate the animal with the following drugs after 5 minutes					
（1）	0.04%Adrenaline	40	0.1		
（2）	0.02%Norepinephrine	20	0.1		
（3）	0.02%Isoproterenol	200	0.1		
3. Observe the effects of β –receptor blockers on blood pressure					
0.1%Timolol		0.1mg/kg	0.1		
Administrate the animal with the following drugs after 5 minutes					
（1）	0.04%Adrenaline	40	0.1		
（2）	0.02%Norepinephrine	200	0.1		

Continued Table

No.		Drug	Dosage (μg/kg)	Drug Volume (ml/kg)	Blood Pressure(mmHg)/ Heart Rate(/min)	
					Before	After
（3）	0.02%Isoproterenol		200	0.1		

4. Observe the effect of cholinergic drugs on blood pressure and cholinergic receptor blockers

No.		Drug	Dosage (μg/kg)	Drug Volume (ml/kg)	Before	After
（1）	0.0002%Ach		2	0.1		
（2）	0.02%Atropine		0.2 mg/kg	0.2		
（3）	0.002%Ach		20	0.1		
（4）	0.02%Ach		200	0.1		

Notes

1. The carotid artery of rats is thinner and shorter than that of the rabbit, therefore you should choose a thinner and rigid tube for arterial intubation.

2. In this experiment, the rat is administered via the artery cannula. However, because the pressure on the three-way opening may cause haemorrhage, you would better dose the rat according to the distal end.

3. The rat's common carotid artery is very thin, and it is difficult to record its blood pressure curve when twisted. Hence, you may adjust the angle between the artery and the catheter, smoothing the blood circulation.

4. The administration volume on rats must not be too large. However, as this study requires multiple administrations, you should inject drugs into the rat supplied with normal saline. You can also formulate corresponding concentrated drugs and dose 0.1 ml of drugs each time.

Other precautions: same as the rabbit experiment.

案例八　传出神经系统药物对家兔血压的影响

知识要求

1.掌握家兔麻醉、手术要点；生物信号采集系统测定血压的方法；血压的形成及影响因素。

2.熟悉传出神经系统药物作用靶点及对血压的影响机制。

能力要求

1.掌握家兔麻醉方法、手术过程及动脉血压测定方法。

2.掌握动物血压测定方法，自行设计相关实验。

3.理解各药物的作用机制，合理解释具体的实验现象。

【实验目的】

学习急性动物麻醉方法、血压测定方法；观察传出神经系统药物对家兔血压的影响及药物间的相互作用，并在受体水平研究药物作用的机制。

【实验原理】

传出神经系统药物涉及面较广，其研究实验方法繁多，血压实验是检验传出神经系统药物及其敏感度的方法，一般采用急性血压实验，动物可采用猫、狗、兔和大鼠。

在研究内容方面，主要围绕神经递质、受体及其效应展开。可采用整体动物实验或离体动物实验，观察药物的效应；还可采用受体拮抗剂作为工具药，判断具体的受体及亚型；利用放射配基结合分析药物与受体的结合作用及结合力大小；还可研究药物对神经递质作用的环节。总之，传出神经系统药物的药理实验很多，具体问题可设计不同的实验来验证。

传出神经系统中的自主神经系统有以乙酰胆碱为递质的副交感神经系统和以去甲肾上腺素为神经递质的交感神经系统，它们互相协调互相对抗，维持机体的生理机能平衡。药物主要影响它们的神经递质和受体，通过受体激动剂或拮抗剂影响动物血压、平滑肌舒张或收缩、腺体分泌等，间接定性分析不同组织、不同部位的受体类型和功能。

动物血压的测定有多种方法，如大鼠尾动脉血压测定法，属于无创测定法，对动物无损伤，可进行多次测量。有创插管生物信号采集系统测定血压所需动物数量少，成本低，可在同一动物样本上测定多种药物，并比较给药前后血压的变化，便于分析药物作用机制。

【实验材料】

1.动物　家兔1只，体重2 kg左右，雄性。

2.药品　生理盐水、500 U/ml肝素钠溶液、2%戊巴比妥钠溶液、0.01%肾上腺素、0.01%去甲肾上腺素、0.05%异丙肾上腺素、1%酚妥拉明、0.1%噻吗洛尔、1%阿托品、乙酰胆碱（0.0001%、0.001%、0.01%）。

3.器材　手术器械（手术刀、手术剪、眼科剪、止血钳、动脉夹），动脉插管，三通管件，血压换能器，注射器（1 ml、5 ml、10 ml），丝线，婴儿秤，兔手术台，手术灯，PowerLab生物信号采集处理系统。

【实验方法与步骤】

1.仪器校准　实验前对仪器进行校准，保存设置文件。具体方法参见PowerLab 7.0使用说明书：记录及分析血压、心室压信号。

2.麻醉　家兔称重后耳缘静脉注射2%戊巴比妥钠1.5 ml/kg，麻醉后仰位固定于手术台。

3.手术　将家兔颈部正中剪毛，切开皮肤，钝性分离浅筋膜，分离气管，做"⊥"形切口，气管插管，粗线结扎固定。继续钝性分离颈部肌肉，在颈部深处找到血管神经鞘，分离出颈总动脉并在下面穿两根丝线，结扎远心端，动脉夹夹闭近心端，用眼科剪尖端在远心端动脉处剪一"V"形斜口。

4.动脉插管　将动脉插管、三通及血压换能器连接并充满500U/ ml肝素钠溶液，检查无气泡后，向心方向插管，丝线结扎固定插管，打开动脉夹，通过三通管件联通血压换能器和动脉插管，观察插管内血液面是否搏动。

5.记录血压曲线　打开PowerLab生物信号采集处理系统，记录一段正常血压曲线，耳缘静脉注射下列药物，给药后立即在软件中标记出相应给药时间点，并记录血压心率变化，每次血压恢复平稳后再给下一药物。

6.结果处理　分析比较药物作用前后血压、心率的变化，分析药物作用机制。

表 2-8-1　传出神经系统药物对麻醉家兔血压的影响

序号	药品	剂量（μg/kg）	给药体积（ml/kg）	血压（mmHg）/心率（/min）	
				给药前	给药后
1. 观察拟肾上腺素药物对血压的影响					
（1）	0.01% 肾上腺素	10	0.1		
（2）	0.01% 去甲肾上腺素	10	0.1		
（3）	0.05% 异丙肾上腺素	50	0.1		
2. 观察 α 受体阻断药对血压的影响					
1% 酚妥拉明		1mg/kg	0.1		
5分钟后给以下列药物					
（1）	0.01% 肾上腺素	10	0.1		
（2）	0.01% 去甲肾上腺素	10	0.1		
（3）	0.05% 异丙肾上腺素	50	0.1		
3. 观察 β 受体阻断药对血压的影响					
0.1% 噻吗洛尔溶液		0.1mg/kg	0.1		
5分钟后给以下列药物					
（1）	0.01% 肾上腺素	10	0.1		
（2）	0.01% 去甲肾上腺素	10	0.1		
（3）	0.05% 异丙肾上腺素	50	0.1		
4. 观察拟胆碱药对血压的影响及胆碱受体阻断药的影响					
（1）	0.0001% 乙酰胆碱	1	0.1		
（2）	1% 阿托品	0.1mg/kg	0.2		
（3）	0.001% 乙酰胆碱	1	0.1		
（4）	0.01% 乙酰胆碱	10	0.1		

【注意事项】

1.家兔麻醉时麻药须缓慢推注，边注射边注意观察其反应，当家兔眼睑反射消失，呼吸、肌肉松弛即停止给药。

2.手术时，除了颈部皮肤经剪刀剪开，其余操作均需钝性分离。

3.寻找家兔颈总动脉前，应先分离出气管，颈总动脉位于气管两侧深处。若未分离气管，不易找到颈总动脉，还易造成其他血管出血。

4.动脉剪"V"形时，血管切勿剪断，但开口也不宜过小，否则难以插入动脉插管。

5.插管前确保血压换能器、三通管件、动脉插管中充满肝素钠生理盐水且无气泡；插管插好后，须保持插管与血管同一直线上，防止插管脱出或弯折影响血压信号记录。

6.因注射药物较多，注意保护耳缘静脉注射部位。

7.某些药物需现用现配，如肾上腺素、乙酰胆碱，否则不能观察到应有的实验现象；因此配制药物之前需仔细阅读药品说明书，保证药物的有效性。

8.每阶段实验后，待血压、心率基本平稳，再进入下一阶段实验。

【思考题】

1.试述肾上腺素、去甲肾上腺素、异丙肾上腺素对心血管作用的异同点。

2.如何验证乙酰胆碱的M样作用和N样作用？

附：传出神经系统药物对大鼠血压的影响

【实验材料】

1.**动物** 大鼠1只，体重400 g左右，性别不限。

2.**药品** 1%戊巴比妥钠或3%水合氯醛溶液、肝素钠，其余药品见表2-8-2。

3.**器材** 手术器械及仪器同家兔实验，动脉插管（自制插管：头皮针针头套入适宜直径的塑料软管制备而成，软管保护动脉避免被针头刺穿）。

【实验方法与步骤】

1.**麻醉** 大鼠称重后，腹腔注射1%戊巴比妥钠0.5 ml/100 g或3%水合氯醛1 ml/100 g，麻醉后仰位固定于手术台。

2.**分离颈总动脉** 手术剪将大鼠颈部正中剪开，用止血钳撕开肌肉层，暴露气管，找到血管神经鞘，钝性分离两侧颈总动脉，分离后动脉下穿两根丝线。

3.**测定血压端动脉插管** 一侧颈总动脉结扎远心端，动脉夹夹闭近心端，用眼科剪尖端在远心端动脉处剪一"V"形斜口。将动脉插管、三通及血压换能器连接并充满500 U/ml肝素溶液，检查无气泡后从远心端向心方向插管，丝线结扎固定插管，打开动脉夹，三通管件联通换能器和动脉插管，观察插管内血液面是否搏动。

4.**给药端动脉插管** 一侧颈总动脉结扎近心端，动脉夹夹闭远心端，用眼科剪尖端在近心端动脉处剪一"V"形斜口。将动脉插管、三通充满500 U/ml肝素溶液，检查无气泡后从近心端向远心方向插管，丝线结扎固定，用于血管内给药。

5.**记录血压曲线** 打开PowerLab生物信号采集处理系统，记录一段正常血压曲线。

6.**给药** 药物经动脉插管给药后，注意补充生理盐水将药物推入血液，同时利用软件记录血压心率变化，每次血压恢复平稳后再给下一药物。

7.**结果处理** 同家兔实验。

表 2-8-2　传出神经系统药物对麻醉大鼠动脉血压的影响

序号	药品	剂量（µg/kg）	给药体积（ml/100g）	血压（mmHg）/心率（/min）	
				给药前	给药后
1. 观察拟肾上腺素药物对血压的影响					
（1）	0.004% 肾上腺素	40	0.1		
（2）	0.02% 去甲肾上腺素	200	0.1		
（3）	0.02% 异丙肾上腺素	200	0.1		
2. 观察 α 受体阻断药对血压的影响					
0.2% 酚妥拉明		2 mg/kg	0.1		
5 分钟后给以下列药物					
（1）	0.004% 肾上腺素	40	0.1		
（2）	0.02% 去甲肾上腺素	200	0.1		
（3）	0.02% 异丙肾上腺素	200	0.1		
3. 观察 β 受体阻断药对血压的影响					
0.1% 噻吗洛尔溶液		0.1 mg/kg	0.1		
5 分钟后给以下列药物					
（1）	0.004% 肾上腺素	40	0.1		
（2）	0.02% 去甲肾上腺素	200	0.1		
（3）	0.02% 异丙肾上腺素	200	0.1		
4. 观察拟胆碱药对血压的影响及胆碱受体阻断药的影响					
（1）	0.0002% 乙酰胆碱	2	0.1		
（2）	0.02% 阿托品	0.2 mg/kg	0.1		
（3）	0.002% 乙酰胆碱	20	0.1		
（4）	0.02% 乙酰胆碱	200	0.1		

【注意事项】

1. 大鼠颈动脉比家兔细且短，动脉插管需选用较细且有一定硬度的插管。

2. 本实验中大鼠给药方式选择颈动脉插管给药，由于向心插管给药时三通开放时易失误造成动物大出血，因此设计给药方向为朝远心端给药，实验成功率会提高很多。

3. 大鼠颈总动脉较细，插管后易发生曲折导致记录不到血压曲线，出现此情况可调整导管与血管的角度，使其顺着血管的方向走行，切勿发生扭曲。

4. 大鼠给药时给药容积不能太大，由于此实验需要连续多次给药，每次还需生理盐水辅助推注药物进入体内，药物剂量也可改为 0.1 ml/ 只，根据给药剂量配制相应浓度的药物。

其他注意事项同家兔实验。

Experiment 9　The Effect of Drugs on Urine Production of Rabbits

Knowledge

1. The method of bladder intubation in rabbits.
2. The process of urine production.
3. The mechanism of drugs in affecting urine production.

Skill

1. Intubate rabbit bladder.
2. Multiple drug administration via rabbit's ear vein.
3. Understand the mechanism of drugs and be able to explain the phenomenon in this study.

Objective

Understand the how to measure the urine production, and observe the effect of drugs on urine production of anaesthetised rabbits.

Background

Urine production includes the filtration of glomeruli and the reabsorption and secretion of renal tubules and collecting ducts.The effective filtration pressure drives the glomerular filtration, mainly depending on glomerular capillary blood pressure, plasma colloidal osmotic pressure and intrasaccular pressure.Usually, the glomerular capillary blood pressure is mainly affected by the arterial pressure. Because of the self-regulation of renal blood flow, glomerular capillary blood pressure is basically stable, unless the blood pressure is lower than 80 mmHg or higher than 180 mmHg. The decrease of plasma colloidal osmotic pressure increases effective filtration pressure and the glomerular filtration rate. Factors that can affect the function of renal tubules and collecting ducts include the solute concentration in renal tubule and antidiuretic hormones.

Methods of evaluating the effect of diuretics on animal experiments include acute and chronic experiments. In acute experiments, we directly collect urine from large animal's ureter or bladder, such as dogs, cats, and rabbits.These experiments only require a short period of time and will not be easily affected by outside factors. However, they need to be performed in non-physiological states, such as anesthesia, and can not provide the same data as the awake state. In chronic experiments, we mainly use metabolic cages to collect urine from rats and mice. These experiments could be carried out under normal physiological states, providing reliable results. However, they are easily affected by temperature or humidity, and their duration can be long.

Diuretics promote the excretion of not only water, but also salts. Therefore, we should also analyse ions in the urine when studying diuretics. We can analyse the mechanism of diuretics by studying the change in the composition of renal tubule fluid, and the effect of the research drug on the activity of various enzymes in kidney tissues by the interception or the micropuncture method, etc.

Furosemide inhibits the reabsorption of chloride and sodium ions at the ascending branch of the medullary loop, affecting the dilution and concentration functions of the kidney with a powerful effect. Hypertonic glucose is an osmotic diuretic that easily metabolised or diffused into tissues, therefore it can only effect for a short period.

Materials

1. Animals: 1 rabbit, weighing about 2 kg, male.

2. Drugs: normal saline, 2% sodium pentobarbital, 6 g/L phenol red, 100 g/L NaOH, 20% glucose, 0.1 g/L norepinephrine, 1% furose mide, pituitrin.

3. Other materials: surgical instruments (such as scalpel, shear, ophthalmic scissor, hemostatic forceps), urinary catheter, syringes (1 ml, 5 ml and 10 ml), threads, rabbit scale, rabbit operating table, operating lamp, and measuring cylinders.

Methods

1. Anesthesia and Fixation

Weigh and fix the rabbits in its supine position, then inject 1.5 ml/kg of 2% pentobarbital.

2. Abdominal Operation

Dehair its abdomen, then make an incision along the midline of the abdomen from the symphysis pubis, and cut open the abdominal cavity along the white line with a scalpel. Avoid damaging other organs. Next, expose the bladder without irritating it, or it may become difficult to intubate.

3. Bladder Cannula

Cut open an incision on the anterior wall where less blood vessels locate, then insert the bladder cannula, avoid tying the ureter. Afterwards, ligate the bladder neck and fasten the cannula. Next, fill the cannula with normal saline with a syringe, and cover the wound with saline gauze.

4. Record 5-minute Normal Urine Output

The count of urine drops in 5 minutes or the volume of urine collected by a beaker.

5. Administrate Drugs and Observe Their Effects

（1）Slowly inject 7 ml/kg of 38℃ normal saline into the rabbit's ear vein, and observe the change of the urine volume.Collect the urine, and continuously record the change of urine volume every 5 minutes for 6 times.

（2）Inject 5 ml of 20% glucose solution intravenously, and continuously record the change of urine volume every 5 minutes for 6 times.

（3）Inject 0.3 ml of 0.1 g/L norepinephrine intravenously, and continuously record the change of urine volume every 5 minutes for 6 times.

（4）Inject 5 mg/kg of furosemide intravenously, and continuously record the change of urine volume every 5 minutes for 6 times.

（5）Inject 0.5 ml of 6 g/L phenol red intravenously, then collect the urine with a petri dish that filled with 100 g/L NaOH. Record the duration before detecting phenol red.

（6）Inject 0.75 U/kg of pituitrin intravenously.

6. Result Processing

Analyse and compare the change of urine volume before and after drug administrations, then analyse the mechanism.Calculate the increased urine volume per unit time by normal saline, glucose and furosemide based on experiment results from the whole class. Afterwards, draw a chart with time as the abscissa, and the increase of urine output as the ordinate. Compare their peak effecting time and the duration of efficacy.

Increased Urine Output = Urine Output per Unit Time after Administration- Urine Output per Unit Time before Administration

Results

Table 2.9.1　The Effect of Drugs on Rabbit's Urine Production

No.	Drug	Dosage （μg/kg）	Administration Volume	Time	Urine Volume （Drops/min）
1.	Normal Urine Volume				
2.	Normal Saline		7 ml/kg	5 min	
				10 min	
				15 min	
				20 min	
				25 min	
				30 min	
3.	20% Glucose	2.5 g/kg	5 ml/kg	5 min	
				10 min	
				15 min	
				20 min	
				25 min	
				30 min	
4.	0.1g/L Norepinephrine		0.3 ml	—	
5.	1% Furosemide	5 mg/kg		5 min	
				10 min	
				15 min	

Continued Table

No.	Drug	Dosage (μg/kg)	Administration Volume	Time	Urine Volume (Drops/min)
				20 min	
				25 min	
				30 min	
6.	Phenol Red		0.5 ml		—
7.	Pituitrin	0.75 U/kg		—	

Notes

1. Feed the rabbit with more vegetables and water before the experiment to increase the basic urine output.

2. Protect the rabbit's ear veins as we will administrate drugs for multiple time in this experiment. Start from tip of its ear, then continuously move the injection site to the root of it.

3. Do not tie up the ureter, or the urine would not be able to enter the bladder.

4. If there is no urine drop for a long time after the drug administration, check if the ureter is twisted or the orifice is lower than the bladder.

5. Do not change the sequence of this experiment. As it's to reduce the urine output based on the increase in urine output, or increase the output based on its reduction.

6. Administrate the next drug after the effect of the previous drug disappears.

Homework

Explain the mechanism of diuretics on urine output.

Appendix: The Effect of Drugs on Urine Production of Rats

Materials

1. Animals: 1 rat, weighing about 400 g, male.

2. Drugs: normal saline, 1% sodium pentobarbital or 3% chloral hydrate, 6 g/L phenol red, 100 g/L NaOH, and other drugs in Tab.2.9.2.

3. Other materials: surgical instruments (such as scalpel, shear, ophthalmic scissor, hemostatic forceps), bladder cannula (scalp needle hose), arterial cannula (experiment 7), syringes (1 ml, 5 ml and 10 ml), threads, rat scale, rat operating table, operating lamp, and measuring cylinders.

Methods

1. Anesthesia and Fixation

Weigh and fix the rat in its supine position, then inject 0.5 ml/kg of 1% pentobarbital or 3% chloral hydrate.

2. Abdominal Operation

Dehair its abdomen, then make an incision along the midline of the abdomen from the symphysis pubis, and cut open the abdominal cavity along the white line with a scalpel. Avoid damaging other organs. Next, expose the bladder without irritating it, or it may become difficult to intubate.

3. Bladder Cannula

Cut open an incision on the anterior wall where less blood vessels locate, then insert the bladder cannula, avoid tying the ureter. Afterwards, ligate the bladder neck and fasten the cannula. Next, fill the cannula with normal saline with a syringe, and cover the wound with saline gauze.

4. Arterial Cannulation

Separate the rat's carotid artery according to experiment 6, then ligate its proximal end. Insert and the fastened arterial cannula toward the distal end. Afterwards, administrate drugs through this cannula.

5. Record 5-minute Normal Urine Output

The count of urine drops in 5 minutes or the volume of urine collected by a beaker.

6. Administrate Drugs and Observe Their Effects

（1）Inject 5 ml of 20% glucose solution, and continuously record the change of urine volume every 5 minutes for 6 times.

（2）Inject 0.3 ml of 0.1 g/L norepinephrine, and continuously record the change of urine volume every 5 minutes for 6 times.

（3）Inject 5 mg/kg of furosemide, and continuously record the change of urine volume every 5 minutes for 6 times.

（4）Inject 0.5 ml of 6 g/L phenol red, then collect the urine with a petri dish that filled with 100 g/L NaOH. Record the duration before detecting phenol red.

（5）Inject 0.75 U/kg of pituitary gland.

7. Result Processing

Analyse and compare the change of urine volume before and after drug administrations, then analyse the mechanism.Calculate the increased urine volume per unit time by normal saline, glucose and furosemide based on experiment results from the whole class. Afterwards, draw a chart with time as the abscissa, and the increase of urine output as the ordinate. Compare their peak effecting time and the duration of efficacy.

Notes

1. Supply the rat with enough water, or give a certain amount of water to it by gavage, to replenish its body fluid.

2. As the administration volume of rats is limited, observe the rat's reaction during the administration and reduce the dosage if necessary.

3. Rats' have less urine output than rabbits, therefore you may appropriately extend the

duration between each administration and urine collection.

Results

Table 2.9.2 The Effect of Drugs on Rat's Urine Production

No.	Drug	Dosage (μg/kg)	Administration Volume	Time	Urine Volume (Drops/min)
1.	Normal Urine Volume				
2.	20% Glucose		0.5 ml	5 min	
				10 min	
				15 min	
				20 min	
				25 min	
				30 min	
3.	0.01% Norepinephrine		0.1 ml	—	
4.	0.1% Furosemide	1 mg/kg	0.1 ml/100 g	5 min	
				10 min	
				15 min	
				20 min	
				25 min	
				30 min	
5.	6 g/L Phenol Red	—	0.5 ml		—
6.	0.36 U/ml Pituitrin	0.75 U/kg	0.1 ml	—	

案例九 药物对家兔尿液生成的影响

知识要求

1.掌握家兔膀胱插管手术方法。

2.熟悉尿液生成过程及影响尿液生成药物的作用机制。

能力要求

1.掌握家兔膀胱插管技术；家兔耳缘静脉多次给药技术。

2.熟悉各药物作用原理，合理解释实验现象。

【实验目的】

了解尿液生成测定实验方法，观察药物对麻醉后兔的尿液生成影响。

【实验原理】

尿液的生成过程包括肾小球的滤过作用及肾小管与集合管的重吸收和分泌作用。肾小球滤过作用的动力是有效滤过压，主要取决于肾小球毛细血管血压、血浆胶体渗透压和囊内压。通常肾小球毛细血管血压主要受全身动脉压的影响，由于肾血流的自身调节作用，肾小球毛细血管血压基本能维持稳定，只有血压低于80 mmHg或高于180 mmHg时，肾小球毛细血管血压才会随血压变化。血浆胶体渗透压降低，会使有效滤过压增加，肾小球滤过率增加。影响肾小管、集合管功能的因素包括改变肾小管液中溶质浓度以及抗利尿激素等。

评价利尿药的动物实验方法包括急性实验和慢性实验。急性实验是直接从输尿管或膀胱收集尿液，适用于大型动物，如狗、猫、家兔等。实验所需时间短，受外界影响小，缺点是需在麻醉或手术等非生理状态下进行，与清醒状态并不完全相同。慢性实验主要采用代谢笼收集尿液。适用于大鼠、小鼠等小型动物，优点是可在动物生理状态下进行实验，所得结果较可靠，缺点是受环境温湿度影响大，实验周期长。

利尿药不仅促进水的排泄，而且也影响盐类的排泄，因此，研究利尿药时还需做尿液的离子分析。分析药物的利尿机制，可通过截留法、微穿刺法等手段，分析各肾小管液组成的变化，研究药物对肾组织中各酶系活性的影响。

呋塞米作用与抑制氯离子和钠离子在髓袢的上行分支的重吸收有关，并影响肾脏的稀释、浓缩功能，有强大的利尿作用。高渗葡萄糖为渗透性利尿药，由于易被代谢或扩散到组织中，利尿作用短暂。

【实验材料】

1. **动物** 家兔1只，体重2 kg左右，雄性。

2. **药品** 生理盐水、2%戊巴比妥钠溶液、6 g/L酚红、100 g/L NaOH、20%葡萄糖、0.1 g/L去甲肾上腺素、1%呋塞米、垂体后叶素。

3. **器材** 手术器械（手术刀、剪毛剪、眼科剪、止血钳），导尿管，注射器（1 ml、5 ml、10 ml），丝线，兔秤，兔手术台，手术灯，小量筒。

【实验方法与步骤】

1. **麻醉及固定** 家兔称重，2%戊巴比妥1.5 ml/kg麻醉，仰卧位固定。

2. **腹部手术** 腹部剪毛，用手术刀从耻骨联合向上沿腹中线作一切口，沿腹白线切开腹腔（注意勿伤及其他内脏器官），暴露膀胱（尽量减少刺激膀胱，防止其缩小，难以插管）。

3. **膀胱插管** 膀胱底两侧辨认输尿管的位置，在前壁血管数量少处切口，插入膀胱插管，用线结扎膀胱颈部，将插管与膀胱用线扎牢固定，用注射器将插管内充满生理盐水，手术完成后用生理盐水纱布覆盖伤口。

4. **记录5分钟正常尿量** 记录5分钟的滴数或用容器收集尿液，测量体积。

5. **给药观察药物作用**

（1）沿耳缘静脉缓慢注入38℃生理盐水7 ml/kg，观察尿量的变化，连续收集尿量，记录尿量随时间的变化（每隔5分钟记录一次，共记录6次）。

（2）静脉注射20%葡萄糖溶液5 ml，记录尿量变化（每隔5分钟记录一次，共记6次）。

（3）静脉注射0.1 g/L去甲肾上腺素0.3 ml。

（4）静脉注射呋塞米5 mg/kg（每隔5分钟记录一次，共记6次）。

（5）静脉注射6 g/L酚红0.5 ml，用盛有100 g/L NaOH溶液的培养皿收集尿液，记录至刚出现酚红所需时间。

（6）静脉注射垂体后叶素0.75 U/kg。

6.结果处理 分析比较药物作用前后尿量的变化，分析药物作用机制；收集全班实验结果，计算给予生理盐水、葡萄糖和呋塞米单位时间内尿量增加量，以时间为横坐标，尿量增加量为纵坐标作图，比较药物作用的高峰时间和作用持续时间。

尿量增加量=给药后单位时间内尿量−给药前单位时间尿量

【实验结果】

表 2-9-1 药物对家兔尿液生成的影响

序号	药品	剂量（µg/kg）	给药体积	时间	尿量（滴/分）
1.	正常尿量				
2.	生理盐水	—	7 ml/kg	5分钟	
				10分钟	
				15分钟	
				20分钟	
				25分钟	
				30分钟	
3.	20% 葡萄糖	2.5 g/kg	5 ml/kg	5分钟	
				10分钟	
				15分钟	
				20分钟	
				25分钟	
				30分钟	
4.	0.1g/L 去甲肾上腺素	30 µg/只	0.3 ml/只	—	
5.	1% 呋塞米	5 mg/kg		5分钟	
				10分钟	
				15分钟	
				20分钟	
				25分钟	
				30分钟	
6.	6 g/L 酚红	—	0.5 ml/只		—
7.	垂体后叶素	0.75 U/kg		—	

【注意事项】

1.实验前给家兔多喂些青菜或水，增加基础尿量。

2.本实验给药次数较多，注意保护耳缘静脉，从耳尖处开始，逐次移向耳根。

3.插管结扎时注意勿将输尿管扎住，防止尿液生成后不能进入膀胱。

4.注射利尿药后若长时间无尿液滴出，应检查输尿管是否扭曲或管口高度高于膀胱。

5.各项实验顺序是按照增加尿量的基础上进行尿量生成减少的实验，尿量减少的基础上进行促进尿量生成的实验，顺序不宜随意变更。

6.待前一药物作用基本消失再注射下一药物。

【思考题】

解释各药物对尿量影响的作用机制。

附：药物对大鼠尿液生成的影响

【实验材料】

1.**动物**　大鼠1只，体重400 g左右，性别不限。

2.**药品**　生理盐水、1%戊巴比妥钠溶液或3%水合氯醛溶液、6 g/L酚红、100 g/L NaOH、其余药品见表2-9-2。

3.**器材**　手术器械（手术刀、剪毛剪、眼科剪、止血钳），自制膀胱插管（头皮针软管），自制动脉插管（见实验七），注射器（1 ml、5 ml、10 ml），丝线，鼠秤，大鼠手术台，手术灯，小量筒。

【实验方法与步骤】

1.**麻醉及固定**　大鼠称重，1%戊巴比妥或3%水合氯醛0.5 ml/100 g腹腔注射进行麻醉，仰卧位固定。

2.**腹部手术**　腹部剪毛，用手术剪从耻骨联合向上沿腹中线纵向剪一小口，用手术镊在腹腔中找到膀胱（尽量减少刺激膀胱，防止其缩小，难以插管）。

3.**膀胱插管**　在膀胱前壁血管少处剪口，将膀胱插管插入膀胱，将其与膀胱颈用线扎牢固定，用注射器将插管内充满生理盐水，完成后用生理盐水纱布覆盖手术切口。

4.**动脉插管**　按照案例八中的方法分离大鼠颈动脉，分离后结扎近心端，动脉插管朝向远心端插入，用丝线扎牢插管与动脉，此插管用于给药。

5.**记录5分钟正常尿量**　记录5分钟滴数或收集尿液，测量体积。

6.**给药观察药物作用**

（1）动脉注射20%葡萄糖溶液5 ml，记录尿量变化（每隔5分钟记录一次，共记6次）。

（2）动脉注射0.1 g/L去甲肾上腺素0.3 ml。

（3）动脉注射呋塞米5 mg/kg（每隔5分钟记录一次，共记6次）。

（4）动脉注射6 g/L酚红0.5 ml，用盛有100 g/L NaOH溶液的培养皿收集尿液，记录刚出现酚红所需时间。

（5）动脉注射垂体后叶素0.75 U/kg。

7.**结果处理**　分析比较药物作用前后尿量的变化，分析药物作用机制；收集全班实验结果，计算给予葡萄糖和呋塞米单位时间内尿量增加量，以时间为横坐标，尿量增加量为纵坐标作图，比较药物作用的高峰时间和作用持续时间。

【注意事项】

1. 大鼠在实验前切勿断水，或于手术前灌胃给予一定量的水，以补充体液。

2. 大鼠的给药容积有限，在给药时应注意观察实验动物对药物的反应，若反应强烈，可减少给药量。

3. 大鼠尿量比家兔少，每次给药后收集尿液的时间可适当延长。

【实验结果】

表 2-9-2　药物对大鼠尿液生成的影响

序号	药品	剂量（µg/kg）	给药体积	时间	尿量（滴／分）
1.	正常尿量				
2.	20% 葡萄糖		0.5 ml/ 只	5 分钟	
				10 分钟	
				15 分钟	
				20 分钟	
				25 分钟	
				30 分钟	
3.	0.01% 去甲肾上腺素		0.1 ml/ 只	—	
4.	0.1% 呋塞米	1 mg/kg	0.1 ml/100g	5 分钟	
				10 分钟	
				15 分钟	
				20 分钟	
				25 分钟	
				30 分钟	
5.	6 g/L 酚红		0.5 ml	—	
6.	0.36 U/ml 垂体后叶素	0.75 U/kg	0.1 ml/ 只	—	

Experiment 10　The Effect of Efferent Nervous System Drugs on Isolated Rabbit Intestines

Knowledge

1. The method of preparing isolated intestines and using Magnus's bath and tension transducer.

2. The distribution of receptor in intestinal muscles, and their diastolic and contractile effects to the intestine.

3. The effect of efferent nervous system drugs on intestines.

Skill

1. Execute rabbits.

2. Prepare isolated intestines, maintain their vitality, and record the intestinal tension.

3. Explain the performance of drugs in this experiment with pharmacology knowledge.

Objective

Understand how to prepare isolated smooth muscles, and obverse effects of efferent nervous system drugs on isolated rabbit intestines.

Methods

Some body tissues can be applied in in-vitro experiments, including: heart, bladder, uterus, trachea, lung, intestine, etc. In vitro studies, the experiment condition are easy to control, the operation is relatively simple, the result are more accurate, and they cost less time. Hence, you may screen a large number of drugs by those studies. However, impure drugs can significantly affect the study result when analysing their mechanisms.

In in-vitro experiments, the study conditions should be controlled to simulate in vivo environment, including temperature around 38℃, 1 to 2 pumps oxygen per second, and a suitable nutrient solution containing certain ions and glucose. Choose specific nutrient solutions for different tissues.

When conducting experiments with isolated intestine tubes, you may choose different parts of them, such as duodenum, jejunum, ileum, due to different study purposes. For example, the small intestine is self-disciplined in a slow frequency, with a starting point located in the duodenum, and the self-discipline weakens from top to bottom. Besides, the jejunum is commonly selected in qualitative experiments, and the ileum is often used in quantitative studies.

This experiment is carried out to study the influence of efferent nervous system drugs on isolated intestinal muscles with the intestine of guinea pigs or rabbits. The guinea pig has less spontaneous ileum activities, providing a stable tracing baseline, and it's sensitive to acetylcholine and cholinergic drugs and may respond them obviously. Hence, it becomes a common method for screening and verifying cholinergic drugs. Besides, the rabbit jejunum has regular oscillating motion, therefore it is suitable for observing the influence of drugs on this motion.

The contraction response of gastrointestinal smooth muscle is mainly controlled by the parasympathetic nerve. Besides, intestinal smooth muscles are rich in cholinergic receptors (M receptors), therefore both M receptor agonists and antagonists can affect the contraction response of smooth muscle. There are mainly α, β, and M receptors in smooth muscles of the rabbit's small intestine. The excitation of α and β receptors can inhibit and relax the small intestine, whereas the excitation of M receptors can excite smooth muscles of the small intestine contract and make it contract.

Drug effects on receptors:1) acetylcholine chloride (Ach): an M receptor agonist that can increase the contraction and peristalsis of the small intestine. 2) atropine (Atro): a competitive M receptor antagonist with no direct effect on intestinal tracts, however it can block the M receptor and resist M-like effects of natural acetylcholine to reduce intestinal contractions. 3) adrenaline (Ad): an α and β receptor agonist that can activate both α and β receptors (mainly the $β_2$ receptor). This activation will dilate the bowel and weakening the movement of small intestine. 4) barium chloride ($BaCl_2$): Ba^{2+} binds to calmodulin in cells, making smooth muscle contract. Besides, Ba^{2+} can also depolarize the cell membrane and cause tonic contraction. However, as $BaCl_2$ does not act by influencing the receptor, atropine cannot counteract this effect.

Materials

1. Animals: a rabbit, male or female.

2. Drugs: $5×10^{-4}$ mol/L acetylcholine chloride, 0.5% atropine sulfate, 0.1% adrenaline hydrochloride (Adr), and 20% $BaCl_2$.

3. Other materials: PowerLab bio-signal recording and analysis system, computer, tension sensor, heat-preserving Magnus's bath, super constant temperature water bath, L-type ventilation hook, high-position infusion bottle, cylinder, beaker, incubator, oxygen cylinder, surgical scissor, ophthalmic scissor, ophthalmology tweezer, sewing needles, cotton threads, syringe, desktop nutrition device, rabbit scale, 1 ml syringe, gavage needle, ruler, etc.

Methods

1. Preparation

Start the software, and turn on the muscle tension measurement function.

2. Adjust the Instrument

Set the temperature of the water bath at $38.5 \pm 0.5\,^{\circ}\mathrm{C}$, add 30 ml Tyrode's solution to the Magnus's bath, then mark the height of liquid inside. Afterwards, introduce 1 to 2 pumps of oxygen per second to the bath.

3. Prepare the Rabbit Intestine Specimen

Execute the rabbit and take out the ileum.Put it into a petri dish that filled with Tyrode's solution, take 1.5 to 2 cm of the ileum, then stitches on both ends of the specimen. Tie an empty knot on one end the thread for an approximately 1 cm small sleeve, and tie a long thread on the other end. Fix the empty knot on the vent hook with a ophthalmic tweezer, then put it into the Magnus's bath, and place the end of the long thread on the other end. Tie an empty knot at the end of the long thread, and hang it on the hook of the tension transducer. Afterwards, adjust the height of the transducer, setting the front load at 1 g, then stabilise the specimen for 20 minutes.

4. Record

Firstly, trace a period of the baseline until it gets stable, then administrate drugs to the rabbit following the order below:

（1）Add 0.2 ml of 5×10^{-4} mol/L acetylcholine chloride into the Magnus's bath, mark the dosing on the computer, then observe the reaction. Turn the system into oscilloscope state with the pause button when the intestine reacts most obviously.

Afterwards, flush the intestine with Tyrode's solution for 3 times to stabilise the specimen for 15 minutes, then add the following drugs.

（2）Turn the system back into the recording state. After having traced a normal curve, add 0.2 ml of 0.5% atropine to the bath and mark it on the computer, then observe the change of this curve. Add 0.2 ml of 5×10^{-4} mol/L acetylcholine chloride after detecting expected effects, then observe the intestinal reaction again. Next, switch the system to pause mode, and flush the intestine for 3 times with Tyrode's solution. Afterwards, stabilise the specimen for 15 minutes.

（3）Switch the system back to the recording state. Add 0.1 ml of 0.01% Adr to the Magnus's bath and mark it on the computer after tracing a normal curve, then observe the curve. Afterwards, turn the computer into pause mode and flush the intestine for 3 times to stabilise the specimen.

（4）Turn the system back into the recording state. After having traced a normal curve, add 0.2 ml of 20% $BaCl_2$ to the bath and mark it on the computer, then observe the change of this curve. Afterwards, switch the system to pause mode and stabilise the specimen. When the baseline get stabilised, add 0.2 ml of 0.5% atropine to the bath and mark it on the computer, then observe the change of this curve. After detecting expected effects, add 0.2 ml of 20% $BaCl_2$ again and observe the intestinal reaction.

5. Result Processing

Print and analyse the bowel contraction curve.

Notes

1. The ileum locates at the end of the small intestine with thin smooth muscle layer and low autonomy. The closer it is to the ileocecal area, the lower its autonomy is, making the baseline more stable.

2. Avoid pulling the intestinal tube, which may reduce its activity.

3. Pay attention to the bath temperature and size of the preload, or it may affect the contraction function of the intestine and its response to the drug.

4. Thread two ends of the intestine by the cross method to avoid twisting the intestine, benefiting the circulation of nutrient solution.

5. Do not close the intestinal cavity when ligating ends of the intestine, otherwise it will affect the drug effect.

6. Flush the intestinal tube for 3 times before each administration, with an interval of 1 minute.

7. As $BaCl_2$ may cause the intestinal tube tonically contract, which is recoverable, so add this drug in final.

8. When administrating drugs, add the solution without touching the thread or the wall of the bath.

9. The specimen may decrease its sensitivity to drugs after taking several high dose of acetylcholine.

Homework

1. What are basic conditions for isolated smooth muscles to maintain their contractile function?

2. Analyse the effect of atropine on intestinal tubes with receptor theory, and discuss the clinical significance of these effects.

3. What does the effect of atropine on the contraction induced by acetylcholine and illustrate?

案例十　传出神经系统药物对兔离体肠管的作用

知识要求

1. 掌握离体肠管的制备方法、麦氏浴槽、张力换能器的使用方法。

2. 熟悉肠管平滑肌的受体分布及对肠管的舒张和收缩活动作用；熟悉传出神经系统药物对肠管的作用。

能力要求

1. 掌握家兔处死方法；离体肠管的制备、保持其活力的方法及肠管张力记录方法。

2. 理解药物的作用机制并能合理解释实验现象。

【实验目的】

掌握离体平滑肌的实验方法。观察传出神经系统药物对家兔离体肠管平滑肌的作用。

【实验原理】

机体的一些组织可以用于离体实验，如心脏、膀胱、子宫、气管、肺、肠等。采用离体实验进行药理实验的特点是：实验条件易于控制、操作简便、结果准确、节省时间，可进行大量药物的筛选。但对药物作用机理分析时，注意不纯的药物可能会对结果产生影响。

当进行离体实验时，必须控制实验条件，模拟体内环境。如控制温度38℃左右；提供氧气：1~2气泡/秒；合适的营养液：含有一定离子和葡萄糖的溶液，不同的组织所选用的营养液不同。

采用离体肠管进行实验，可根据实验目的不同进行选择小肠的不同部位（十二指肠、空肠、回肠）。例如小肠具有自律性：特点是频率较慢，起搏点位于十二指肠，自律性自上而下渐弱；空肠多用于定性实验，回肠多用于定量实验。

本次实验研究传出神经系统药物对离体肠肌收缩活动的影响，一般采用豚鼠或家兔的肠管。豚鼠回肠自发活动少，描记基线稳定，对乙酰胆碱和拟胆碱药敏感，反应明显，是筛选、检定拟胆碱药的常用实验方法。家兔空肠因具有规则的摆动运动，适用于观察药物对此运动的影响。

胃肠道平滑肌的收缩反应主要由副交感神经控制，肠道平滑肌富含M受体，M受体激动剂和拮抗剂均可明显影响平滑肌的收缩反应。家兔小肠平滑肌上主要存在α受体、β受体、M受体。α受体、β受体的兴奋可使小肠平滑肌抑制而舒张；M受体的兴奋可使小肠平滑肌兴奋而收缩。

药品对受体的作用：①氯乙酰胆碱：M受体激动剂，使小肠收缩幅度增加，蠕动加强。②阿托品：M受体拮抗剂，为竞争性拮抗剂，单独用药对肠管无直接作用，可阻断M受体，对抗乙酰胆碱的M样作用，使肠管收缩幅度降低。③肾上腺素：α受体、β受体激动剂，可激活α受体、β受体（主要是 β_2 受体），α受体、β受体激动可产生与M受体激动相反的效应，表现为肠管舒张，小肠蠕动减弱。④氯化钡：Ba^{2+} 进入细胞与钙调蛋白结合，使平滑肌收缩；Ba^{2+} 可使细胞膜发生去极化。所以加入 $BaCl_2$ 后肠管会发生强直性收缩，$BaCl_2$ 并非作用于受体，所以阿托品不能对抗这一作用。

【实验材料】

1.动物及药品　家兔，雌雄不限；5×10^{-4} mol/L 氯乙酰胆碱；0.5% 硫酸阿托品；0.1% 盐酸肾上腺素；20% $BaCl_2$。

2.仪器设备及手术器械等　PowerLab生物信号记录分析系统、计算机、张力传感器、保温式麦氏浴槽、超级恒温水浴、"L"型通气钩、高位吊瓶、量筒、烧杯、培养器、氧气瓶、外科剪刀、眼科剪刀、眼科镊子、缝合针、棉线、注射器、台式营养器、兔秤、1ml注射器、灌胃针、标尺等。

【实验方法与步骤】

1.调试仪器　在电脑上打开软件，选择进入肌张力测定状态。

2.调节仪器 将超级恒温水浴温度调至 38.5 ± 0.5 ℃，向麦氏浴槽中加入 30 ml 台氏液，标记液面高度，通入氧气（1~2个气泡/秒）

3.制备家兔肠管标本 处死家兔，打开腹腔，取出回肠，放入盛有台式液的培养皿内，取回肠 1.5~2 cm，将肠管标本两端用缝针各穿一线，一端打一空结（约 1 cm 的小套），另一端穿上长线打结，用眼科镊钳住空结固定于通气钩上，放入麦氏浴槽中，将另一端长线的尽端打一空结，挂在张力换能器的小钩上，调节换能器高度，使前负荷为 1 g，稳定标本 20 分钟。

4.记录 先描记一段基线至平稳状态，然后按下列顺序给药。

（1）向麦氏浴槽内加入 5×10^{-4} mol/L 氯乙酰胆碱 0.2 ml，同时在软件中作给药标记，观察肠段反应。当反应最明显时，用暂停键，将计算机转入"示波状态"。用台氏液冲洗肠管 3 遍，稳定标本 15 分钟，加入下列药物。

（2）将系统重新转入"记录状态"，描记一段正常曲线后，向麦氏浴槽中加 0.5% 阿托品 0.2 ml 并作标记，观察曲线变化，出现预期作用后加 5×10^{-4} mol/L 氯乙酰胆碱 0.2 ml，观察肠段反应。系统转为"暂停"，用台氏液冲洗肠管 3 遍。稳定标本 15 分钟。

（3）将系统重新转入"记录状态"，描记一段正常曲线后向麦氏浴槽中加 0.01% 盐酸肾上腺素 0.1 ml 并作标记，观察曲线变化。将计算机转入"暂停"下冲洗肠管 3 次，稳定标本。

（4）将系统重新转入"记录状态"，描记一段正常曲线后，向麦氏浴槽中加 20% $BaCl_2$ 0.2 ml 并作标记，观察曲线变化。将计算机转入"暂停"下冲洗肠管，稳定标本，基线稳定后，加入 0.5% 阿托品 0.2 ml 并作标记，观察曲线变化，出现预期作用后加 20% $BaCl_2$ 0.2 ml，观察肠段反应。

5.结果处理 打印肠管收缩曲线，分析原因。

【注意事项】

1.回肠位于小肠的末端，平滑肌层较薄，自律性低，越靠近回盲部自律性越低，基线越平稳。

2.操作时应避免牵拉肠管，造成肠管活性降低。

3.注意控制浴槽水温与前负荷的大小，否则影响肠段的收缩功能及对药物的反应。

4.肠管两端穿线采用十字交叉法，肠管不易扭曲，便于营养液的流通。

5.结扎肠两端时切忌扎闭肠腔，否则影响药物作用强度。

6.每次给药前均应冲洗肠管 3 次，中间间隔 1 分钟。

7. $BaCl_2$ 使肠管产生强直性收缩，不能恢复，所以最后加 $BaCl_2$。

8.给药时将药液直接加入药液，不要碰线，也不要碰壁。

9.本标本在使用几次大剂量乙酰胆碱后可能会失去敏感性。

【思考题】

1.离体平滑肌保持其收缩功能需要哪些基本条件？

2.试从受体学说分析阿托品对肠管的作用，并讨论这些作用的临床意义。

3.阿托品对乙酰胆碱和 $BaCl_2$ 引起收缩反应的影响说明了什么？

Experiment 11　The Therapeutic and Toxic Effect of Cardiac Glycosides on Rabbits' Heart

Knowledge

1. The method of replicating heart failure model.
2. Keypoints of ventricular intubation.
3. Methods of judging cardiac function.
4. Therapeutic and toxic effects of cardiac glycosides and their mechanisms.
5. The clinical application of cardiac glycosides.

Skill

1. Replicate heart failure models.
2. Ventricularly intubate rabbits.
3. Measure the rabbit's heart function.
4. Understand the significance of cardiac function indicators.
5. Understand the mechanism of drugs and be able to explain the phenomenon in this study.

Objective

Study the replication of heart failure models. Understand the significance of cardiac function indicators. Observe the therapeutic and toxic effects of cardiac glycosides on animal heart failure.

Background

The heart pumping function, including stroke volume, stroke work, ejection fraction, and heart index, etc., in animal experiments illustrates the systematic performance of myocardial contractility, preload and afterload functions. The evaluation of cardiac hemodynamics and overall cardiac function is one of the most important part in studying cardiovascular drugs, and all cardiovascular drugs must be evaluated with this method. Through these researches, we may understand the effect of drugs on myocardial function and peripheral blood vessels.

Heart failure is a clinical syndrome caused by reduced myocardial contractility and cardiac output because of various reasons, with the symptoms of reduced cardiac output, increased end-diastolic pressure, abnormal myocardial diastolic performance, decreased arterial blood pressure, and increased venous blood pressure.

Sodium pentobarbital can inhibit the uptake of calcium by the sarcoplasmic reticulum of cardiomyocytes and increase the binding of calcium ions with the sarcoplasmic reticulum phosphate, reducing calcium ions in cardiomyocytes and causing negative inotropic effects. It may lead to heart failure in the final. Cardiac glycosides have obvious effects on calcium deficiency heart failure, however they have limited safety range and may also cause poisoning and arrhythmia.

Observes the change in heart functions caused by heart failure, and cardiac glycoside treatment and poisoning through cardiac hemodynamic parameters.

Related indicators and their significance in this experiment

1. Left ventricular systolic pressure (LVSP): the left systolic ventricular pressure. The LVSP increases when the preload, afterload or the myocardial contractility increases.

2. Left ventricular end diastolic pressure (LVEDP): represents the left ventricular preload. It is an important parameter for analysing cardiac function.

3. The maximum increase and decrease rate of left ventricular pressure ($LV \pm d_p/d_{t_{max}}$): reflects the change of the ventricular wall tension to evaluate diastolic functiona certain extent, with $+ d_p/d_{t_{max}}$ to evaluate the systolic function, and $- d_p/d_{t_{max}}$ for the maximum rate of contractile component extension during the myocardial diastole.

4. Blood pressure (BP): including systolic blood pressure (SAP), diastolic blood pressure (DAP), and mean arterial pressure (MAP).

5. Heart rate (HR): the count of heartbeats per minute.

Materials

1. Animals: 1 rabbit, weighing about 2 kg, male.

2. Drugs: normal saline, 500 U/ml sodium heparin, 3% sodium pentobarbital, 20% urethane, 0.0125% convolvulin K.

3. Other materials: PowerLab biosignal recording and analysis system, micro syringe pump, surgical instruments, arterial cannula, ventricular cannula, rabbit scale, syringe, etc.

Methods

1. Rabbit Anesthesia

Weigh and fix the rabbit on the operating table with its supine position, then intravenously inject it with 5ml/kg of 20% urethane in the ear vein.

2. Neck Surgery

Dehair its neck coat, cut open the skin of its neck centre, and bluntly separate the carotid arteries on both sides (refer to Experiment 8).

3. Tracheal Intubation

Intubate the trachea and connect it to the ventilator.

4. Arterial Cannulation

Fill the arterial cannula with sodium heparin saline for left carotid artery cannulation, and connect it to the system to measure its blood pressure (refer to Experiment 8). Record the normal blood pressure, and perform ventricular intubation after the blood pressure stabilises.

5. Ventricular Cannulation

Measure the ventricular pressure by the right common carotid artery. Remove the arterial clip when the cannula enters the artery, then slowly push it into the left ventricle through the aortic valve. When the lower edge blood pressure wave reach around 0 mmHg and looks flat at the diastolic peak, the catheter has entered the left ventricular cavity. If the waveform remains unchanged when you push another 0.2 to 0.4cm, you can fix the cannula and measure the ventricular pressure through it.

6. Record Normal Heart Function Indicators

Heart rate (HR), blood pressure (BP), left ventricular systolic pressure (LVSP), left ventricular end diastolic pressure (LVEDP), left ventricular mean pressure (LMVP), the maximum rate of increase and decrease of left ventricular pressure (LV $d_p/d_{t_{max}}$), etc.

7. Establish the Acute Heart Failure Model

After heparinised the rabbit, slowly inject the rabbit with 20 mg/kg of 2% sodium pentobarbital intravenously until the left ventricular pressure drops to 30% to 40% of it before the administration. This is the index of acute heart failure.

8. Cardiac Glycoside Therapy

Infuse 6 ml of 0.125 mg/ml convolvulin K through the rabbit's ear vein at a constant rate with a injection pump. Record the change of indicators during the infusion.

9. Result Processing

Intercept real-time recording curve and collect corresponding data with the software. Analyse and compare the change of various indicators before and after the model building, and before and after the cardiac glycoside treatment, then analyse the mechanism of drugs in this experiment.

Results

Table 2.11.1　Therapeutic and Toxic Effects of Cardiac Glycosides on Rabbit's Heart

	LVSP (mmHg)	LVEDP (mmHg)	LMVP (mmHg)	LV $d_p/d_{t_{max}}$ (mmHg/s)	HR (bpm)	BP (mmHg)
Before Modeling						
Heart Failure Model						
Cardiac Glycoside Therapy						
Cardiac Glycoside Poisoning						

Notes

1. Pay attention to the depth of the ventricular intubation.Measure the length of the cannula before intubation.Be gentle and keep observing the change of blood pressure during the process. When feel resistance, draw back the tube for 2 to 3mm.

2. Sodium pentobarbital is an anaesthetic that may cause respiratory depression.Therefore, use a ventilator in this experiment to prevent excessive anesthesia and suffocation.

3. The tolerable amount of sodium pentobarbital varies among individuals, therefore the dosage should be flexible.

4. You may also judge whether the rabbit's poisoned by detecting the arrhythmia by the 2-lead electrocardiogram.

Homework

Describe the cardiotonic mechanism of cardiac glycosides. What effect may excessive cardiac glycosides cause on heart?

案例十一　强心苷对兔心衰的治疗作用与毒理作用

知识要求

1.掌握心衰模型复制方法，心室插管要点，心功能测定方法。

2.熟悉强心苷的药理、毒理作用及机制。

3.了解强心苷药物的临床应用。

能力要求

1.掌握心衰模型的复制，家兔心室插管及心功能测定方法。

2.理解心功能指标意义，熟知药物的作用机制并能合理解释实验现象。

【实验目的】

学习心衰模型的复制；掌握心脏功能指标意义；观察强心苷药物对动物心衰的治疗及毒性作用。

【实验原理】

整体动物实验中心脏泵血功能（心搏量、搏功、射血分数、心脏指数等）是心肌收缩能力、前、后负荷综合作用的表现。心脏的血流动力学和整体心功能评价是研究心血管药物的重要环节，所有心血管药物都要进行这方面评价。通过血流动力学研究，可了解药物对心肌功能和外周血管的影响。

心衰是由多种病因造成心肌收缩力降低、心排出量减少的一种临床综合征，具体表现为：心排出量减少、舒张末期压力增高、心肌舒缩功能异常、动脉血压下降、静脉血压增高。

戊巴比妥钠可抑制心肌细胞肌浆网对钙离子的摄取，并增加肌浆网磷酸酯对钙离子的结合，使心肌细胞内钙离子减少，产生负性肌力作用导致心衰。强心苷对心脏缺钙引起的心衰治疗效果明显，但其使用时安全范围小，容易发生中毒，引起各种心律失常。

本实验通过心脏血流动力学指标参数，观察心衰、强心苷治疗及中毒的相关心功能变化。

【本实验相关指标及意义】

1.左心室收缩压力（LVSP） 等容收缩期左心室压力，当前后负荷升高或心肌收缩力加强时，LVSP升高。

2.左室舒张末期压（LVEDP） 代表左室前负荷，是分析心功能的重要参数。

3.左室内压最大上升和下降速率（LV ± $d_p/d_{t_{max}}$） 一定程度上反映室壁张力的变化速率，$+d_p/d_{t_{max}}$用于评价收缩功能，反映心肌舒张时收缩成分延长的最大速度；$-d_p/d_{t_{max}}$用于评价舒张功能。

4.血压（BP） 包括收缩压（SAP）、舒张压（DAP）、平均动脉压（MAP）。

5.心率（HR） 每分钟心跳次数。

【实验材料】

1.动物 家兔1只，体重2 kg左右，雄性。

2.药品 生理盐水、500 U/ml 肝素钠溶液、3%戊巴比妥钠溶液、20%乌拉坦溶液、0.0125%毒毛旋花子苷K溶液。

3.仪器设备及手术器械 PowerLab生物信号记录分析系统、微量注射泵、手术器械、动脉插管、心室插管、兔秤、注射器等。

【实验方法与步骤】

1.家兔麻醉 家兔称重，20%乌拉坦以5 ml/kg剂量沿耳缘静脉注射麻醉，仰卧位固定于手术台。

2.颈部手术 剪去颈部被毛，沿颈部正中切开皮肤，分离气管及两侧颈动脉（可参考案例八）。

3.气管插管 气管插管，连接呼吸机。

4.动脉插管 动脉插管充满肝素钠生理盐水进行左侧颈动脉插管，连接通道用于测定血压（可参考案例八）。记录正常血压，待血压稳定后进行心室插管。

5.心室插管 右侧颈总动脉用于测定心室压，插管进入动脉后，移去动脉夹，缓慢推进，使其通过主动脉瓣到达左心室，当血压波变成下沿达 0 mmHg附近，具有明显舒张期峰顶平坦的波形时，表明导管进入左室腔内，若再送入0.2~0.4 cm，还保持同样波形，即可结扎固定，该通道用于测定心室压。

6.记录正常心功能指标 心率（HR）、血压（BP）、左室收缩压（LVSP），左室舒张末期压（LVEDP），左室平均压（LMVP），左室内压最大上升和下降速率（LV $d_p/d_{t_{max}}$）等。

7. 建立急性心衰模型　当家兔全身肝素化后，将2%戊巴比妥钠溶液以20 mg/kg的剂量缓慢静脉注射，待左心室压下降至给药前的30%~40%，此为急性心衰指标。

8. 强心苷治疗　0.125 mg/ml毒毛花苷K经微量注射泵由耳缘静脉恒速输注（一般输入6 ml）。输注过程记录各指标变化情况。

9. 结果处理　实验结果可以截取实时记录曲线并通过软件采集相应数据。分析比较造模前后、强心苷治疗前后各指标变化，分析药物作用机制。

【实验结果】

表 2-11-1　强心苷对家兔在体心脏的药理与毒理作用

	LVSP （mmHg）	LVEDP （mmHg）	LMVP （mmHg）	LV $d_p/d_{t_{max}}$ （mmHg/s）	HR （bpm）	BP （mmHg）
造模前						
心衰模型						
强心苷治疗						
强心苷中毒						

【注意事项】

1. 判断心室插管的深度：插管前可先测量长度，插管时宜动作轻柔，插管时边插边观察血压变化，如遇到阻力，可回抽2~3 mm。

2. 戊巴比妥钠为麻醉药，可引起呼吸抑制，因此本实验应使用呼吸机，以避免动物麻醉过度窒息而死。

3. 引起心衰的戊巴比妥钠量因个体差异而不同，实验中应灵活掌握。

4. 实验中也可测定 Ⅱ 导联心电图，以心律失常为指标判断是否中毒。

【思考题】

强心苷的强心作用机制是什么？过量强心苷对心脏的影响有哪些？

Experiment 12   The in vitro Effect of Drugs on Tumour Cell Proliferation

Knowledge

1. The MTT method.

2. Keypoints of screening anti-tumour drugs.

3. Basic methods of cell experiments.

4. The pharmacological effects and mechanisms of anti-tumour drugs.

Skill

1. Basic operation skills of cell experiment.

2. Measure the cell proliferation by the MTT method.

3. Calculate the IC_{50} of anti-tumour drugs and design related experiments.

Objective

Measure cell proliferation by the MTT method and calculate the IC_{50} of anti-tumour drugs.

Background

We usually carry out preliminary anti-tumour drug screening by in-vitro experiments. If a drug can inhibit the proliferation of human or animal tumour cells, further study may be deployed. In vitro experiments are simple and short-term, and only require a small amount of medicine, therefore the drug can be screened at a high throughput. However, in vitro experiments cannot reflect some actual features of drugs, such as pharmacodynamic, pharmacokinetic, and toxicity characteristics. Therefore, its results require verification by in vivo experiments.

MTT (methyl thiazolyl tetrazolium) is a water-soluble powder that can be reduced into water-insoluble blue-purple crystal formazan by the succinate dehydrogenase in mitochondria of only living cells. Hence, the scale of living cells is correlated with the amount of formazan. Furthermore, formazan can be dissolved with DMSO (dimethyl sulfoxide) to form a blue-violet solution. We can measure its colour with a microplate reader to detect its OD value and figure out the concentration of formazan, reflecting the number of living cells. Therefore, we can determine the inhibitory effect of drugs on tumour cells and calculate its IC_{50}.

Materials

1. Cell lines: human hepatic cancer cell line HepG2.

2. Drugs: vincristine sulfate, DMEM medium, fetal bovine serum, trypsin solution, MTT, dimethyl sulfoxide (DMSO), PBS (pH7.4) (phosphate buffer solution).

3. Other materials: carbon dioxide incubator, purified workbench, desktop centrifuge, microplate reader, inverted microscope, cell counting plate, sterile 96-well culture plate, pipette, sterile centrifuge tube, alcohol lamp, alcohol cotton ball, etc.

Methods

1. Cell Culture

Culture the cell in a DMEM medium containing 10% fetal bovine serum in a 5% CO_2, 37°C cell incubator after the resuscitation. Renew the medium every other day, then passage the cell when they grow into 70%~80% confluence.

2. Cell Seeding

Digest cells with trypsin until they just fall off, then terminate the DMEM medium. Collect the cell to prepare a suspension and count them. Next, adjust the concentration to 5U/ml and inoculate them in a 96-well plate, 200 μl per well. Afterwards, place them in a cell culture then incubate overnight.

3. Drug Treatment

Discard the medium when cells adhere to the wall, then add drugs prepared with the complete medium to the cell. The drug concentration are listed as follows: 0.125 μg/ml, 0.25 μg/ml, 0.50 μg/ml, 1.00μg/ml, 2.00 μg/ml, 4.00 μg/ml, 8.00 μg/ml, 16.00 μg/ml and 32.00 μg/ml. Add complete medium into the control group. Set each concentration with 6 wells, and incubate them for 48 hours.

4. Cell Count Assay

Add 20 μl of 5 mg/ml MTT solution to the cell and incubate them for 4 hours. Discard the medium in the well, then add 150 μl of DMSO solution to each well and shake well for 10 minutes. Afterwards, measure the absorbance at 490 nm with a microplate reader.

$$\text{Growth Inhibition Rate:} GI = \left(1 - \frac{\text{OD Value of the Drug Group}}{\text{OD Value of the Control Group}}\right) \times 100\%$$

Use GI and drug concentration to calculate IC_{50} by SPSS.

Results

Table 2.12.1　Effects of Drugs on the Proliferation of Human Hepatic Cancer Cell Line HepG2

Drug	Concentration	OD Value	Inhibition Rate of Each Well	$\overline{X} \pm SD$

Notes

1. Aseptic operation during cell experiments.

2. Accurately prepare drugs, and add cells and reagents.

Homework

What are the advantages and disadvantages of in vitro experiments for anti-tumour drugs? Do they have clinical applications?

案例十二　药物体外对肿瘤细胞增殖的影响

知识要求

1.掌握MTT法测定原理及方法；抗肿瘤药物筛选方法要点。

2.熟悉细胞基本操作实验方法及要点；抗肿瘤药物的药理作用及机制。

能力要求

1.掌握细胞实验基本操作技能及MTT法测定细胞增殖的实验方法。

2.了解抗肿瘤药物IC_{50}的计算方法及设计相关实验。

【实验目的】

学习MTT法体外测定药物抗肿瘤生长的作用及IC_{50}的计算。

【实验原理】

抗肿瘤药物的初步筛选通常先采用体外实验进行，若药物在体外可以抑制人或动物肿瘤细胞的增殖，则可进行深入研究。体外实验方法简便，周期短，用药量少，可高通量筛选药物。但体外实验脱离了机体的整体性，不能反映出实际药效、药代动力学、毒性等方面的情况，所以，体外实验还需体内实验的进一步验证。

甲基噻唑基四氮唑（MTT）是黄色粉末，可溶于水，在活细胞中被线粒体琥珀酸脱氢酶还原为水不溶性的蓝紫色结晶甲臜，由于死细胞不含琥珀酸脱氢酶，不会产生甲臜，因此，甲臜的产生量与活细胞的数量呈正相关。甲臜结晶可溶于二甲基亚砜（DMSO）成为蓝紫色溶液，其溶液颜色深浅可用酶标仪检测OD值，反映活细胞的数目。根据此原理可检测药物对肿瘤细胞生长的抑制作用并计算IC_{50}值。

【实验材料】

1.细胞株及药品　人肝癌细胞株HepG2，硫酸长春新碱，DMEM培养基，胎牛血清，胰蛋白酶溶液，MTT，二甲基亚砜（DMSO），PBS（pH7.4）（磷酸盐缓冲溶液）。

2.**其他材料** 二氧化碳培养箱，净化工作台，台式离心机，酶标仪，倒置显微镜，细胞计数板，无菌96孔培养板，移液器，无菌离心管，酒精灯，酒精棉球等。

【实验方法与步骤】

1.**细胞培养** 细胞复苏后用含10%胎牛血清的DMEM培养基于5%CO_2，37℃细胞培养箱中培养，隔天换液，待细胞生长至70%~80%汇合度时进行传代。

2.**细胞接种** 胰蛋白酶消化至贴壁细胞刚好脱落，DMEM培养液终止消化，收集细胞制备成细胞悬液，细胞计数，调整细胞数5×10^4个/ml，接种于96孔板，每孔200 μl，置于细胞培养箱培养过夜。

3.**药物处理** 细胞贴壁后，将旧培养基弃去，用完全培养基配制不同浓度的药物后加入细胞中，药物浓度分别为0.125 μg/ml，0.25 μg/ml，0.50 μg/ml，1.00 μg/ml，2.00 μg/ml，4.00 μg/ml，8.00 μg/ml，16.00 μg/ml，32.00 μg/ml，阴性对照组加入不含药物的完全培养基，每个浓度设6个复孔，培养箱中孵育48小时。

4.**测定结果** 细胞中加入5 mg/ml MTT溶液20 μl，继续孵育4小时。弃去孔内培养液，每孔加DMSO溶液150 μl，震荡摇匀10分钟，酶标仪490 nm测定吸光度。

5.**数据处理** 计算各组吸光度值平均值和标准差；根据下列公式计算抑制率：

$$生长抑制率公式: GI（生长抑制率）=\left(1-\frac{药物组OD值}{阴性对照组OD值}\right)\times100\%$$

以生长抑制率和对应药物浓度利用SPSS软件（logi法）计算IC_{50}。

【实验结果】

表2-12-1 药物对人肝癌细胞株HepG2增殖的影响

药物	浓度	OD值	各孔抑制率	$\overline{X}\pm SD$

【注意事项】

1.细胞操作过程注意无菌操作。

2.药物配制浓度、向96孔板内加细胞及试剂时加样体积要精确。

【思考题】

抗肿瘤药物的体外实验方法有哪些优缺点和实际应用？

第三篇
基础临床药理学自主实验设计典型案例

Chapter 3

Basic Clinical Pharmacology Experiments

Experiment 1 Influencing Factors of Type A Adverse Drug Actions

Knowledge

1. Understand the basic principles and main factors of adverse drug reactions.
2. Understand factors that may cause or influence drug effects or interactions.

Skills

1. Be proficient in basic experiment skills, including gripping mouse and drug administration.
2. Understand how to apply statistic methods in designing experiments.
3. Systematically analyse experiment results utilizing statistic methods.

Objective

1. Understand the role of adverse drug reactions in clinical practice by observing drug interactions in this experiment, especially the tape atoxic reaction.
2. Review gripping mice, intraperitoneal and subcutaneous injections.

Background

Type A adverse drug reactions are also known as dose-related adverse reactions，which caused by the drug itself or its metabolites, and the inherent pharmacological effect is enhanced or sustained. It is dose-dependent and predictable, with a high incidence, but low risk, low mortality, and large individual susceptibility differences. Type A adverse drug reactions are related to factors such as age, gender, and pathological state, including drug side effects, toxic effects, and secondary reaction, first-dose effect, after-effects, etc. Among them, different doses of drugs, routes of administration, drug interactions and changes in drug metabolism in vivo are the key factors leading to the occurrence of such adverse reactions. This case focuses on the verification basic research on the above factors.

Experiment 1.1 Effects of Sodium Pentobarbital on Mice at Different Dosages

Knowledge

1. The influence of drug dosage on its effects; judgment criteria of righting reflection; methods for analysing quantitative data.

2. Pharmacological effects of pentobarbital sodium; keypoints of mice grouping, numbering and intraperitoneal injection.

Skill

1. Mice grouping, numbering and intraperitoneal injection.

2. Understand the significance of observation indicators in experiments and explain the phenomenon in the experiment with pharmacology knowledge.

3. Accurately record and manage the quantitative and qualitative data with statistical methods.

Objective

Understand the relationship between dosage and drug effects by observing the varied efficacy and toxicity of sodium pentobarbital at different doses on mice.

Background

Pentobarbital sodium is a sedative drug that can cause effects ranged from sedation, hypnosis to anesthesia with the increasing dosage.

Materials

1. Animals: 3 mice, weighing from 18 to 22 g, male or female.

2. Drugs: 0.2%, 0.4% and 0.8% sodium pentobarbital solution.

3. Other materials: rat scale, 1 ml syringe, picric acid, etc.

Methods

1. Weigh and number 3 same-gender and similar-weighed mice, then observe their normal

activities.

2. Intraperitoneally inject 0.1 ml/10g of 0.2%, 0.4% and 0.8% sodium pentobarbital solution, respectively, to all mice.

3. Immediately record the administration time and observe mice's activity. Record the time that the righting reflex disappears and recovers in time and manage these data in Tab. 3.1.1.

4. Carry out a statistical analysis based on experiment results from the whole class, then analyse and summarise the study result.

Results

Table 3.1.1   Influences of Dosage on the Effect of Intraperitoneally Administered Sodium Pentobarbital in Mice

No.	Weight (g)	Dose (mg/kg)	Time of Administration	Disappearance Time of Righting Reflex	Recovery Time of Righting Reflex	Time of Taking Effect (min)	Duration (min)
1							
2							
3							

Notes

1. Choose similar weighed mice to reduce individual differences.

2. Carefully observe mice's reactions after the administration, and record each time point with a stopwatch to avoid bias.

Homework

1. What's the relationship and clinical significance between drug dosage and its effects?

2. What type of drug reaction is it in this experiment?

Experiment 1.2 The Influence of Administration Routes on Drug Effects

Knowledge

1. The influence of administration route on drug effects.

2. Judgment criteria of mice's central excitement level.

3. Methods of analysing quantitative and qualitative data.

4. Pharmacological effects of nikethamide.

5. Keypoints of mice grouping, numbering and drug administration.

Skill

1. Mice grouping, numbering and drug administration; accurately judge mice's central excitement level.

2. Explain the reaction of central excitement with pharmacology knowledge.

3. Accurately record and manage the quantitative and qualitative data with statistical methods.

~ · ~ ·

Objective

Compare the influence of administration routes on drug effects.

Background

Nikethamide is a central stimulant that can cause excitement, convulsions and even death in animals, whereas different administration routes affect the effect speed and degree of this drug. It can also cause different reactions on different animals at the same dose.

Materials

1. Animals: 3 mice, weighing from 18 to 22 g.

2. Drugs: 2% nikethamide solution.

3. Other materials: rat scale, 1 ml syringe, gastric applicator, picric acid, etc.

Methods

1. Weigh and number 3 same-gender similar-weighed mice, then observe their normal activities

2. Administrate 0.2 ml/10g of 2% nikethamide solution to mice by intraperitoneal, subcutaneous and gavage injections, respectively.

3. Immediately record the administration time and observe mice's activity. Record the time that the mouse shows vertical tail, jump, and convulsion or death, and manage these data in Tab. 3.1.2.

4. Carry out a statistical analysis based on experiment results from the whole class, then analyse and summarise the study result.

Results

Table 3.1.2   Influences of Administration Routes on the Effect of Nikethamide in Mice

No.	Weight (g)	Administration Route	Time of Administration	Time of Vertical Tail	Time of Jump	Time of Convulsion or Death	Incubation Duration (min)
1							
2							
3							

Notes

1. Choose similar-weighed mice to reduce individual differences.

2. Carefully observe mice's reactions after the administration, and record each time point with a stopwatch to avoid bias.

3. Mice can be very excited after the administration, therefore you should place them in separate and covered cages immediately after the injection.

Homework

1. What's the influence of drug administration routes on its effects? Explain the mechanism of this phenomenon.

2. According to this study, what should be paid attention to during the administration in clinical practice?

Experiment 1.3 Drug Interactions

Knowledge

1. The synergy and antagonism between drugs.

2. Pharmacological effects of neostigmine, streptomycin, succinycholine.

Skill

1. Mice grouping, numbering and intraperitoneal injection.

2. Understand drug interactions and explain them with pharmacology knowledge.

3. Accurately record and manage the quantitative and qualitative data with statistical methods.

Objective

Understand the synergy and antagonism between drugs.

Background

When drugs are used together, interactions may occur in terms of pharmacodynamics or pharmacokinetics, leading to changes in drug effects. Common drug interactions includes: efficacy enhancement or reduction, side effects enhancement or reduction, and other irrelevant effects. We prefer enhanced efficacy and weakened toxicity in clinical practices, and should avoid the weakened efficacy or enhanced side effects.

Streptomycin is an aminoglycoside antibiotic with significant ototoxicity and nephrotoxicity, especially under the condition of clinical therapeutic doses. Succinycholine is a commonly used depolarized muscle relaxant that has a significant peripheral neuromuscular blocking effect, and generally maintains a short duration and recovers quickly. Neostigmine is a cholinesterase inhibitor that can effectively enhance the peripheral tone of the parasympathetic nerve and relieve muscle weakness, but cannot be used for poisoning relief except for polarized muscle relaxants.

Materials

1. Animals: 6 mice, weighing from 18 to 22 g, male or female.

2. Drugs: neostigmine 0.5 mg/kg, streptomycin sulfate 630 mg/kg, succinycholine 2.5 mg/kg, normal saline.

3. Other materials: rat scale, 1 ml syringe, picric acid, etc.

Methods

1. Weigh and number 6 same-gender similar-weighed mice, then observe their normal activities.

Mouse 1: blank control, intraperitoneal injection of equal volume of normal saline.

Mouse 2: intraperitoneal injection of streptomycin sulfate 630 mg/kg.

Mouse 3: intraperitoneal injection of succinylcholine 2.5 mg/kg.

Mouse 4: intraperitoneal injection of streptomycin sulfate 630 mg/kg, followed by injection of succinycholine 2.5 mg/kg after 2 min.

Mouse 5: intraperitoneal injection of streptomycin sulfate 630 mg/kg, followed by injection of neostigmine 0.5 mg/kg after 2 min.

Mouse 6: intraperitoneal injection of succinylcholine 2.5 mg/kg, followed by injection of neostigmine 0.5 mg/kg after 2 min.

2. Observe and record the response of each group of mice within 15 min after administration, including breathing, color of the mucosa of the lips, death, and compare final results. Record mice's reactions in Table 3.1.3.

3. Carry out statistical analysis based on experiment results from the whole class, then analyse and summarise the study result.

Results

Table 3.1.3　Results of Drug Interactions

No.	Weight (g)	The First Administration		The Second Administration		Results of Drug Interactions
		Drug	Reactions	Drug	Reactions	
1						
2						
3						
4						
5						
6						

Notes

1. Synchronize injections as much as possible, and design parallel experiments to reduce systematic errors.

Homework

1. How many types of adverse drug interaction reactions are there?
2. What does the experiment illustrate? What is its clinical significance?

Experiment 1.4　The Influence of Hepatic Drug–Metabolising Enzymes on Drug Effects

Knowledge

1. The significance of hepatic drug-metabolising enzymes in pharmacology.

2. Hepatic drug-metabolising enzyme inhibitors and inducers; understand the effects of phenobarbital sodium and cimetidine on hepatic drug-metabolising enzymes.

3. The influence of hepatic drug-metabolising enzyme inhibition and induction on the effect of pentobarbital sodium.

Skill

1. Mice grouping and numbering, and replication of liver drug-metabolising enzyme induction and inhibition models.

2. Accurately record the result and manage it with statistical methods, then analyse the phenomenon in this experiment.

~ • ~ • ~ • ~ • ~ • ~ • ~ • ~ • ~ • ~ • ~ • ~ • ~ • ~ • ~ • ~ • ~ • ~ • ~

Objective

Understand the influence of hepatic drug-metabolising enzyme on drug effects.

Background

The hepatic drug-metabolising enzyme is an important system for drug metabolism in animal body. Most drugs get inactivated or activated through this system, therefore its activity affects drug actions.

Some substances can induce the expression of hepatic drug-metabolising enzymes, or increase their stability, therefore we classify them as hepatic drug-metabolising enzyme inducers. There are also some inhibitors that could inhibit the activity of this system or enzyme-mediated reactions. While using these drugs, we must pay attention to their effects on liver drug enzymes. Besides, we should also comprehensively consider the possible interaction when use them with other drugs in combination.

Phenobarbital sodium is a liver drug enzyme inducer, whereas cimetidine is a hepatic drug-metabolising enzyme inhibitor. As pentobarbital sodium is mainly inactivated by liver metabolism, changes in liver drug enzyme system will influence its effects.

Materials

1. Animals: 3 mice, weighing from 18 to 22 g, male or female.

2. Drugs: 0.75% phenobarbital, 0.2% cimetidine, 0.2% pentobarbital sodium, normal saline

3. Other materials: rat scale, 1 ml syringe, picric acid, etc.

Methods

1. Group 3 mice into normal control, inducer and inhibitor group, respectively, then intraperitoneally inject them with 0.1ml/10g of normal saline, 0.75% phenobarbital, and 0.2% cimetidine solutions, respectively, for 2 to 3 days before the experiment.

2. Intraperitoneally inject 0.1 ml/10g of 0.2% pentobarbital sodium to all mice in the study, and record their disappearance and recovery time of the righting reflex in Tab. 3.1.4.

3. Carry out statistical analysis based on experiment results from the whole class, then analyse and summarise the study result.

Results

Table 3.1.4   The Influence of Hepatic Drug–Metabolising Enzyme Inhibitor and Inducer on the Effect of Pentobarbital Sodium

Group	Weight (g)	Time of Administration	Disappearance Time of Righting Reflex	Recovery Time of Righting Reflex	Duration of Incubation (min)	Duration of efficacy (min)
Normal Control						
Inhibitor						
Inducer						

Notes

1. Group mice randomly to reduce individual difference between groups by balancing their weights.

2. Accurately record the time about mice's righting reflex.

Homework

What influence do of hepatic drug-metabolising enzyme inducer and inhibitor have on drug effects?

What should be paid attention to when use drugs that may induce or inhibit the hepatic drug-metabolising enzyme system in clinical practice?

案例一   药物 A 型不良反应发生因素研究

知识要求

1.理解药物不良反应发生基本原理与主要因素。

2.理解药物相互作用发生基本因素。

能力要求

1.掌握小鼠的捉拿、给药等动物实验基本技能操作。

2.掌握药物不良反应发生原因及实验设计方法。

3.掌握生物统计学方法分析实验结果。

【实验目的】

1. 观察药物不良反应的发生，了解其主要影响因素，特别是药物相互作用后产生的 A 型毒性反应，以加深理解药物不良反应发生原因与临床意义。

2. 复习巩固基础药理学实验部分小鼠的捉拿、腹腔、皮下注射方法。

【实验原理】

A型药物不良反应又称为剂量相关性不良反应。是由药物本身或其代谢物所引起，为固有药理作用增强或持续所致。具有剂量依赖性和可预测性，发生率较高，但危险性小，病死率低，个体易感性差异大，与年龄、性别、病理状态等因素有关，包括药物的副作用、毒性作用以及继发反应、首剂效应、后遗效应等。其中药物作用不同剂量、给药途径、药物相互作用以及体内药物代谢变化是导致该类不良反应发生的关键因素。本案例着重就以上因素进行验证基础研究。

实验一　不同剂量戊巴比妥钠对小鼠作用的影响

知识要求

1. 掌握药物剂量对药物作用的影响；翻正反射的判断标准；定量反应分析方法。

2. 熟悉戊巴比妥钠的药理作用；小鼠的分组、编号及腹腔注射要点。

能力要求

1. 掌握小鼠随机分组、编号及腹腔注射等操作。

2. 理解实验观察项目指标的意义，应用药理学知识解释实验现象。

3. 正确记录定量反应、定性反应数据并进行统计分析。

【实验目的】

通过观察不同剂量戊巴比妥钠对小鼠作用的影响，了解药物剂量与作用的关系。

【实验原理】

戊巴比妥钠为镇静催眠药物，依剂量递增其作用表现为镇静、催眠及麻醉作用。

【实验材料】

1. **动物**　小鼠3只，体重18~22 g，雌雄不限。

2. **药品**　0.2%、0.4%、0.8%戊巴比妥钠溶液。

3. **其他材料**　鼠秤、1 ml注射器、苦味酸等。

【实验方法与步骤】

1. **分组**　取性别相同，体重相近的小鼠3只，称重、编号，观察一般活动，然后给药。

2. **给药**　分别腹腔注射0.2%、0.4%、0.8%戊巴比妥钠溶液0.1 ml/10 g。

3. **观察指标**　给药后立即记录给药时间，观察小鼠活动情况，及时记录小鼠翻正反射消失及恢复时间。按表3-1-1记录原始数据并处理结果。

4. **结果处理**　实验结束后，对全班实验结果进行统计分析，分析实验结果并得出结论。

【实验结果】

表 3-1-1   腹腔注射不同剂量戊巴比妥钠对小鼠作用的影响

编号	体重（g）	药物剂量（mg/kg）	给药时间	翻正反射消失时间	翻正反射恢复时间	作用开始时间（分钟）	作用维持时间（分钟）
1							
2							
3							

【注意事项】

1.小鼠体重宜相近，减少个体差异。

2.仔细观察小鼠给药后的表现，及时用秒表记录各时间点，避免误差太大。

思考题

1.了解药物剂量与作用的关系及其临床意义。

2.本实验属于哪种药物反应类型？

实验二   不同给药途径对药物作用的影响

知识要求

1.掌握不同给药途径对药物作用的影响；小鼠中枢兴奋的程度及判定指标；定量反应、定性反应数据的分析方法。

2.熟悉尼可刹米的药理学作用；小鼠的分组、编号及不同给药途径操作要点。

能力要求

1.掌握小鼠随机分组、编号及各不同给药途径的给药方法；准确把握中枢兴奋判定指标，完成数据记录。

2.理解中枢兴奋的表现，能应用药理学知识解释实验现象。

3.正确记录定量反应、定性反应数据并进行统计分析。

【实验目的】

比较给药途径对药物作用的影响。

【实验原理】

尼可刹米为中枢兴奋药，可引起动物兴奋、惊厥或死亡。不同给药途径影响药物进入体内的速度及程度，相同剂量下引起动物的反应亦不同。

【实验材料】

1.动物   小鼠3只，体重18~22 g，雌雄不限。

2.药品 2%尼可刹米溶液。

3.其他材料 鼠秤、1 ml注射器、灌胃器、苦味酸等。

【实验方法与步骤】

1.分组 取性别相同，体重相近的小鼠3只，称重、编号，观察一般活动，然后给药。

2.给药 分别采用腹腔注射、皮下注射、灌胃给以小鼠2%尼可刹米溶液0.2 ml/10 g。

3.观察指标 给药后立即记录给药时间，观察小鼠活动情况，及时记录小鼠出现竖尾、跳跃、惊厥或死亡的时间，计算药物作用潜伏期。将结果记录于表3-1-2。

4.结果处理 实验结束后，对全班实验结果进行统计分析，分析实验结果并得出结论。

【实验结果】

表 3-1-2 尼可刹米不同给药途径对小鼠作用的影响

编号	体重（g）	给药途径	给药时间	竖尾时间	跳跃时间	惊厥或死亡时间	作用潜伏期（min）
1							
2							
3							

【注意事项】

1.小鼠体重宜相近，减少个体差异。

2.仔细观察小鼠给药后的表现，及时记录各时间点，应精确到秒，避免误差太大。

3.小鼠给药后较为兴奋，给药后的小鼠与未给药小鼠应分笼放置，且给药后立即将小鼠置于有盖的鼠笼中，防止小鼠窜出。

思考题

1.不同给药途径对药物作用产生哪些影响？原因是什么？

2.在临床给药过程中，应注意什么？

实验三 药物效应的协同与拮抗作用

知识要求

1.掌握药物的协同与拮抗作用原理。

2.熟悉链霉素、琥珀胆碱和新斯的明的药理学作用。

能力要求

1.掌握小鼠随机分组、编号及不同给药方法。

2.理解药物之间的相互作用关系，应用临床药理学知识解释实验现象。

3.正确记录定量反应、定性反应数据并进行统计分析。

【实验目的】

认识药物的协同与拮抗作用。

【实验原理】

药物合用时，可能会在药效学或药动学方面发生相互作用，导致药物的作用发生改变。药物之间的相互通常作用表现为：药效作用加强、药效作用减弱、毒副作用增强、毒副作用减弱。通常临床中希望出现药效作用增强、毒副作用减弱，避免药效作用减弱、毒副作用增强的效果。

链霉素是氨基糖苷类抗生素，具有明显的耳毒性和肾毒性，特别是在临床治疗剂量条件下会出现明显的神经肌肉阻滞作用。琥珀胆碱是一种常用的去极化型肌肉松弛剂，具有显著的外周神经肌肉阻断作用，一般作用维持时间较短，恢复迅速。新斯的明是胆碱酯酶抑制剂，可有效增强副交感神经的外周张力，缓解肌无力现象，但不能用于去极化型肌肉松弛剂的中毒解救。

【实验材料】

1. 动物　小鼠6只，体重18~22 g；

2. 药品　新斯的明0.5 mg/kg、硫酸链霉素630 mg/kg、琥珀胆碱2.5 mg/kg、生理盐水；

3. 其他材料　电子秤、1 ml注射器、苦味酸等。

【实验方法与步骤】

1. 分组　取性别相同，体重相近的小鼠6只，称重、编号，观察一般活动，然后分别予以以下不同处理：

小鼠1：空白对照，腹腔注射等体积生理盐水；

小鼠2：腹腔注射硫酸链霉素630 mg/kg；

小鼠3：腹腔注射琥珀胆碱2.5 mg/kg；

小鼠4：先腹腔注射硫酸链霉素630 mg/kg，2分钟后注射琥珀胆碱2.5 mg/kg；

小鼠5：先腹腔注射硫酸链霉素630 mg/kg，2分钟后注射新斯的明0.5 mg/kg；

小鼠6：先腹腔注射琥珀胆碱2.5 mg/kg，2分钟后注射新斯的明0.5 mg/kg；

2. 给药并观察指标　给药后观察记录小鼠反应，观察15分钟并记录各组表现：肌张力、呼吸情况、口唇黏膜颜色、死亡情况，比较最终结果；将结果记录于表3-1-3。

3. 结果处理　实验结束后，对全班实验数据进行统计分析，分析实验结果并得出结论。

【实验结果】

表3-1-3　药物的相互作用结果

编号	体重（g）	第一次给药		第二次给药		相互作用的结果
		药剂	反应	药剂	反应	
1						
2						
3						

续表

编号	体重 （g）	第一次给药		第二次给药		相互作用的结果
		药剂	反应	药剂	反应	
4						
5						
6						

【注意事项】

尽量做到同步注射，设计平行实验减少系统误差。

思考题

1.药物相互作用不良反应有几种类型？

2.本次实验说明什么问题？其临床意义如何？

实验四　肝药酶对药物作用的影响

知识要求

1.掌握肝药酶在药理学中的意义。

2.熟悉肝药酶抑制剂和诱导剂的含义；了解苯巴比妥钠、西咪替丁对肝药酶的作用。

3.理解肝药酶抑制模型和诱导模型对戊巴比妥钠作用的影响。

能力要求

1.掌握小鼠随机分组及复制肝药酶诱导、抑制模型的方法。

2.正确处理实验结果并进行统计分析，合理分析实验现象。

【实验目的】

通过实验了解肝药酶代谢的变化对药物作用的影响。

【实验原理】

肝药酶是体内药物代谢的重要酶系，药物经肝药酶代谢失活或活化，因而肝药酶的活性可影响药物对机体的作用。

一些化学物质可诱导肝药酶的表达或增加其稳定性，称为肝药酶诱导剂；还有一些物质可抑制肝药酶的活性或抑制酶介导的反应，称为肝药酶抑制剂。在服用这些化学物时应注意对肝药酶的影响，与其他药物合用时，更要综合考虑对肝药酶的影响及其他药物作用的改变。

苯巴比妥钠为肝药酶诱导剂，西咪替丁为肝药酶抑制剂。戊巴比妥钠经肝脏代谢后会失活，肝药酶活性的改变将影响其药物作用。

【实验材料】

1.**动物**　小鼠3只，体重18~22 g，雌雄不限。

2.**药品**　0.75%苯巴比妥溶液，0.2%西咪替丁溶液，0.2%戊巴比妥钠溶液，生理盐水。

3.**其他材料**　鼠秤、1ml注射器、苦味酸等。

【实验方法与步骤】

1.**分组**　小鼠3只，分为正常组、肝药酶诱导组、肝药酶抑制组，实验前分别每天腹腔注射一次生理盐水、0.75%苯巴比妥溶液、0.2%西咪替丁溶液0.1 ml/10 g，注射2~3天。

2.**给药并观察指标**　实验时，3只小鼠腹腔注射0.2%戊巴比妥钠溶液 0.1 ml/10 g，记录翻正反射消失和恢复时间。

3.**结果处理**　实验结果记录于表3-1-4。对全班实验结果进行统计分析，分析实验结果并得出结论。

【实验结果】

表 3-1-4　肝药酶抑制剂、肝药酶诱导剂对戊巴比妥钠作用的影响

组别	体重（g）	给药时间	翻正反射消失时间	翻正反射恢复时间	作用潜伏期（分钟）	作用维持时间（分钟）
正常组						
肝药酶抑制组						
肝药酶诱导组						

【注意事项】

1.注意小鼠诱导之前按体重随机分组，减少各组间个体差异。

2.观察翻正反射时注意将各时间点记录准确。

思考题

肝药酶活性改变对药物作用的影响是什么？临床用药时应注意什么？

Experiment 2　The Influence of Pathological Conditions on Drug Effects

Knowledge

1. Influences of pathological hepatic and renal conditions on drug effects.
2. The modelling principle and method of liver and kidney pathological models.
3. Keypoints of normal and pathological morphology of liver and kidney.

Skill:

1. Mice grouping and numbering, replicate mouse hepatic and renal injury models.
2. Understand the effect of liver disease on pentobarbital sodium and kidney injury on Streptomycin, and be able to explain these effects with pharmacology knowledge.
3. Correctly collect, observe and analyse liver and kidney samples.

Objective

Observe the influence of liver and kidney injuries on drug effects

Background

Liver is an important metabolic organ in animal body. Most drugs are metabolised by the liver into inactive or less-active compounds. In case of liver injury and weakened metabolic capacity, drug effects maybe increased or weakened. Carbon tetrachloride is a hepatotoxic compound and can induce toxic hepatitis models in animal models, therefore we may use it to observe the influence of liver damage on drug effects and discover liver-protecting drugs.

Pentobarbital is mainly eliminated by liver metabolism, and the rate of elimination varies from liver functional state to liver, and it is possible to produce toxic reactions at safe doses.

Kidney is an important excretion organ in animal body. Furthermore, some drugs are metabolised by the kidney. When the renal function is damaged, the drug excretion would be slowed down, leading to drug accumulations and enhanced effects. Mercury chloride is a kidney toxicant that its mechanism of causing renal failure is stated as follows: Hg^{2+} can be reabsorbed by renal tubules after being filtered by glomerulus, then combining with sulfhydryls

(SH) and disulfides in renal tubular epithelial cells, affecting the intracellular enzyme activities and eventually leading to increased renal tubule permeability and blockage of renal tubules, causing anuria and oliguria. In addition, the original urine may leak to the renal interstitium, causing edema and oppressing renal tubules, then leading to acute renal failure.

In this kidney damage model, the animal's renal blood flow is decreased, with the increased Scr and BUN level. Their 24-hour creatinine clearance rate and 24-hour total creatinine and urea nitrogen excretion are increased as well. The animal suffers significant oliguria first, followed by polyuria, and various proteins in their urine. When observe their kidneys by naked eye, you may find significantly enlarged renal tissues, increased renal index, renal cortex ischemia, and medulla congestions. Using a microscope, you may also fine degenerated and necrotic renal proximal tubule cells.

Streptomycin is a kidney-toxic aminoglycoside antibacterial agent that mainly excreted through the kidney. When renal insufficiency occurs and the excretion of this drug is reduced, it is very likely to cause toxicity.

Materials

1. Animals: 4 mice, weighing from 18 to 22 g; 4 rats, weighing from 220 to 250 g, male or female.

2. Drugs: 5% carbon tetrachloride oil solution, 200 mg/kg gentamicin solution, 0.3% sodium pentobarbital, 250 mg/kg streptomycin solution.

3. Other materials: rat scale, 1 ml syringe, picric acid, etc.

Methods & Results

1. The Influence of Liver Injury on the Effect of Pentobarbital Sodium

（1）Group and number 4 mice into pathological and normal control group, 2 mice in each group. Subcutaneouslyinject 0.1 ml/10g of 5% carbon tetrachloride oil solution to mice in the pathological group 48 hours before the experiment, inducing liver injury models.

（2）Those in the normal control group will receive blank oil solvent.

（3）During the experiment, all mice will be injected intraperitoneally with 0.1 ml/10g of 0.3% sodium pentobarbital. Record the time of mice's righting reflex disappears and recovers in Table 3.2.1.

（4）Execute the mouse after experiment, then compare their liver tissue.

Table 3.2.1   The Influence of Liver Injury on the Effect of Pentobarbital Sodium

No.	Weight (g)	Dosage (mg/kg)	Time of Administration	Disappearance Time of Righting Reflex	Recovery Time of Righting Reflex	Time of Taking Effect (min)	Duration (min)
Injury 1							
Injury 2							
Control 1							
Control 2							

2. The Influence of Renal Injury on the Effect of Kanamycin

（1）Group and number 4 rats into pathological and normal control group, 2 mice in each group. Intraperitoneally inject 200mg/kg of gentamicin solution to mice in the pathological group 72 hours before the study, inducing renal injury models.

（2）Those in the normal control group will receive normal saline.

（3）During the experiment, all mice will be injected intraperitoneally with streptomycin 250 mg/kg to observe the animal reactions (muscle tone, respiratory conditions, oral and lip mucosa color, death) to compare the final results. Record mice's reactions in Table 3.2.2.

（4）Execute the mouse after experiment, then compare their kidney tissue.

Table 3.2.2　The Influence of Renal Injury on the Effect of Kanamycin

No.	Weight (g)	Dosage (mg/kg)	Time of Administration	Reactions	Pathological Observations
Injury 1					
Injury 2					
Control 1					
Control 2					

Notes

1. Dilute the carbon tetrachloride with peanut oil or soybean oil and make them fully dissolved stirred.

2. Fast the mouse overnight after the injection of carbon tetrachloride for severer liver damage.

3. Keep the room temperature at 24 to 25℃, and keep the mice warm. Otherwise the metabolism of mice would be slowed down and they would be difficult to wake up, if it is too cold.

4. Take liver and kidney of mice after the experiment. Compared the liver from injury group to those from the normal group, the damaged liver should be enlarged, and some of them would be greyish-yellow, congested, and greasy for touch.Their lobules will be clearer than normal ones. The damaged kidney will be obviously enlarged, and you may find its cortex paler and its medulla more congested under longitudinal section.

Homework

1. What influence does liver function have on pentobarbital sodium? Why? Which kind of drugs are susceptible to liver function?

2. What influence does kidney function have on pentobarbital kanamycin? Why? Which kind of drugs are susceptible to renal function?

3. What should be paid attention to when prescribing drugs that are susceptible to liver and kidney function in clinical practice?

案例二　病理因素对药物效应的影响

知识要求

1.掌握肝、肾病理状态下对药物作用的影响。

2.掌握肝、肾病理模型的造模原理及方法。

3.了解肝脏、肾脏正常及病理组织形态学变化要点。

能力要求

1.掌握小鼠随机分组、编号及复制肝病、肾病模型的方法。

2.掌握采集肝脏、肾脏样本的方法，观察并比较形态、结构。

3.理解肝病对戊巴比妥钠、肾病对链霉素作用的影响，应用药理学知识解释实验现象、分析结果。

【实验目的】

观察肝肾疾病对药物作用的影响。

【实验原理】

肝脏是体内重要的代谢器官，绝大部分药物经过肝脏代谢，代谢产物为无活性或活性产物，肝功能损伤后，代谢能力减弱，引起相应药物活性增强或减弱。四氯化碳是一种细胞毒性物质，能迅速被肝脏吸收，对肝脏造成毒性作用，致使肝细胞坏死，破坏肝功能，常用于观察肝脏对药物作用的影响及筛选保肝药物研究。

戊巴比妥能够经肝脏代谢而被消除，肝脏功能状态的不同对其消除的速率不同，极有可能在安全剂量下产生毒性反应。

肾脏主要参与药物的排出，有些药物还经由肾脏代谢。肾功能损伤时，主要影响药物排出，导致药物蓄积，造成药物作用增强。高剂量的庆大霉素具有显著的肾毒性，可致使肾小管细胞坏死，肾小管通透性增加、肾小管堵塞，导致无尿、少尿，从而诱发急性肾衰。模型特点：肾血流量下降，Scr水平升高，BUN水平升高，24小时肌酐清除率显著降低，24小时肌酐、尿素氮总排出量减少。动物首先出现少尿，随后出现多尿，尿中有蛋白及各类管型。肉眼观察，肾组织明显肿大，肾指数增加，肾皮质缺血，髓质淤血。镜下观察，肾近曲小管细胞变性坏死。

链霉素属于氨基糖苷类抗菌药，主要经肾脏排泄，具有肾毒性，肾功能不全时药物排出减少，更易导致动物中毒。

【实验材料】

1.动物　小鼠4只，体重18~22 g；大鼠4只，体重220~250 g，均雌雄不限。

2.药品　5%四氯化碳油溶液，200 mg/kg庆大霉素溶液，0.3%戊巴比妥钠，250 mg/kg链霉素溶液。

3.其他材料　鼠秤、1 ml注射器、苦味酸等。

【实验方法与步骤】

1.肝功能损伤对戊巴比妥钠作用的影响

（1）取小鼠4只，分成两组（病理模型组和正常对照组）每组2只。病理模型组于实验前72小时皮下注射5%四氯化碳油溶液0.1 ml/10 g，造成肝脏损伤。

（2）正常对照组皮下注射等量的油溶剂。

（3）实验时两组动物均腹腔注射0.3%戊巴比妥钠溶液0.1 ml/10 g，记录翻正反射消失和恢复时间于表3-2-1。

（4）实验结束后，处死动物，取病理组与正常组动物的肝组织进行比较。

表3-2-1　小鼠肝功能损伤对戊巴比妥钠作用的影响

组别编号	体重（g）	药物剂量（mg/kg）	给药时间	翻正反射消失时间	翻正反射恢复时间	作用开始时间（分钟）	作用维持时间（分钟）
病理组1							
病例组2							
正常组1							
正常组2							

2.肾功能损伤对链霉素作用的影响

（1）取大鼠4只，分成两组（病理模型组和正常对照组）每组2只。病理模型组于实验前72小时腹腔注射庆大霉素溶液200 mg/kg，造成肾脏功能损伤。

（2）正常对照组腹腔注射等量的生理盐水。

（3）实验时两组动物均皮下注射链霉素250 mg/kg，观察动物反应（肌张力、呼吸情况、口唇黏膜颜色、死亡情况）比较最终结果。将结果记录数据于表3-2-2。

（4）实验结束后，动物安乐死处理，将病理组与正常组动物的肾组织进行比较。

表3-2-2　小鼠肾功能损伤对链霉素作用的影响

组别编号	体重（g）	链霉素（mg/kg）	给药时间	动物反应	病理学观察肾组织
病理组1					
病例组2					
正常组1					
正常组2					

【注意事项】

1.四氯化碳用油（花生油或豆油）稀释成所需浓度，且须充分搅拌使其完全溶解，注射剂量不宜过大，否则易造成动物中毒死亡。

2.四氯化碳注射后须禁食过夜，肝损伤效果显著。

3.室温宜控制在24~25℃，若室温低，小鼠麻醉后应给予保暖措施，否则代谢减慢，不易苏醒。

4.实验结束后取小鼠肝脏、肾脏。与正常组相比，肝脏损伤组小鼠肝脏肿大，有的充血或呈灰黄色，触之有油腻感，其小叶比正常肝脏更清楚；肾脏损伤组肾脏明显肿大，纵切后，可见皮质部较苍白，髓质部有充血。

思考题

1.肝脏功能对戊巴比妥钠产生什么影响？为什么？哪些药物易受肝脏功能影响？

2.肾功能对链霉素作用产生什么影响？为什么？ 哪些药物易受肾脏功能影响？

3.易受肝肾功能影响的药物在临床用药时应注意什么？

Experiment 3   Determination of Pharmacokinetic Parameters of Sodium Salicylate

Knowledge

1. The significance and calculation methods of pharmacokinetic parameters; blood sampling and its processing methods of rabbit.

2. Pharmacokinetic process of salicylate sodium.

Skill

1. Blood sampling from rabbits, and prepare the plasma.

2. Accurately determine pharmacokinetic parameters according to the concentration-time curve.

3. Design experiments to determine pharmacokinetic parameters of drugs.

Objective

Understand how to determine pharmacokinetic parameters, including plasma half-life, apparent distribution volume and clearance rate, and the significance of this process.

Background

Pharmacokinetic is a subject that studies the in vivo process of drugs, usually with mathematical models and pharmacokinetic parameters, playing an important role in evaluating new drugs. By monitoring the pharmacokinetic process of a drug, we can predict its efficacy and toxicity, ameliorate its clinical use, provide guidance for the rational use of it, and benefit its individual use.

Most drugs are eliminated following the first-order kinetic process. The relationship between the log value of plasma drug concentration and time after (*i.v.*) injection is:

$$\lg C_t = \lg C_0 - \frac{k}{2.303} t \quad (3.3.1)$$

Hence, $t_{1/2} = 0.693/k$ (by hour or minute) (3.3.2)

Measure the plasma drug concentration of some time points, and draw an appropriate straight line according to these points, then calculate the slope (*s*) of this straight line.

Calculate the elimination rate constant according to the formula $k=-2.303×s$ （3.3.3）

Then figure out the $t_{1/2}$ according to the formula (3.3.2).

Apparent distribution volume, V_d, means the required blood volume when all the administrated drug uniformly distributes in the body, reaching the initial plasma drug concentration C_0.

$$V_d = \frac{\text{Intravenously Administrated Dosage (mg/kg)}}{C_0} \quad \text{(ml/kg or L/kg) (3.3.4)}$$

Clearance rate (CL) refers to the volume of blood that body removes all the drug within it per unit time.

$$CL = \frac{0.693}{t_{1/2}} × V_d \quad (\frac{ml}{min}/kg) \quad (3.3.5)$$

The method to determine the concentration of salicylate sodium: salicylic acid forms a purple complex with ferric chloride in acidic environments, and this complex shows an optical density at a wavelength of 520nm, which is directly proportional to its concentration.

Materials

1. Animals: a rabbit, weighing around 2.5 kg, male or female.

2. Drugs: 10% sodium salicylate, 0.06% standard sodium salicylate, 10% ferric chloride, 10% trichloroacetic acid, 0.5% heparin, normal saline, and xylene.

3. Other materials: rabbit fixing box, heparinised test tube, 10 ml centrifuge tube, 5 and 1 ml pipette and pipette tips, 5 ml syringe, #6 gauge needles, spectrophotometer, centrifuge, vortex mixer, surgery blade, marker, dry cotton ball, disposable glove, beaker, xylene.

Methods & Results

1. Blood Sampling

Sample blood with a heparinised test tube. Weigh the rabbit and fix it in a rabbit box, then remove the coat on its both ear veins. Stimulate one of its ear veins with xylene, then cut it and sample 3ml of blood in a test tube as the control. Shake the blood well to prevent clotting. Press a cotton ball on the rabbit's ear to stop bleeding.

2. Drug Administration and Blood Sampling

Slowly inject 150 mg/kg of 10% sodium salicylate into the other ear vein, then take blood from at the 1, 3, 5, 10, 15, 20, 30, 45, and 60 minute. Take 3 ml of blood in different tubes and shake them well, then let stand to separate the plasma.

3. Determine the Content of Sodium Salicylate in Blood Samples

Add samples and reagents into centrifuge tubes as it's shown in the table below. Fully mix the content in each tube with the vortex mixer, then centrifuge them for 10 minutes at 2000 rpm. Afterwards, take 3 ml of the supernatant from each tube and add them to another set of clean tubes, then add 0.3 ml of 10% ferric chloride into each tube, and mix well to develop colour. Next, measure their OD values at 520 nm with a spectrophotometer. Record the result in Tab. 3.3.1.

Table 3.3.1　Results of Sodium Salicylate Determination in Blood Samples

No.	10% Trichloroacetic Acid (ml)	Plasma (ml)	0.06% Sodium Salicylate (ml)	Normal Saline (ml)	OD (520 nm)
Control	4	1	0	1	
Standard	4	1	1	0	
1 min	4	1	0	1	
3 min	4	1	0	1	
5 min	4	1	0	1	
10 min	4	1	0	1	
15 min	4	1	0	1	
20 min	4	1	0	1	
30 min	4	1	0	1	
45 min	4	1	0	1	
60 min	4	1	0	1	

4. Results Processing

According to the concentration calculated with the OD value, draw a concentration-time curve, with time as the abscissa and logarithmic concentration as the ordinate. Figure out and CL with formula 3.3.2 to 3.3.5. When calculating the C_0, you may extend the concentration-time line to the vertical axis, and the antilog of is the intersection point of this line and the vertical axis.

Notes

1. No leakage in intravenous administrations to ensure accurate dosage.

2. Do not use the same vein for administration and blood sampling.

3. If possible, collect blood within a minute. You may also take blood from the carotid artery.

4. Accurately record the time of blood collections.

5. Figure out the drug concentration with OD values by the regression equation for accurate results.

Homework

1. Will the duration of drug administration and blood collection influence the result of the experiment? Why?

2. What will drug leakage cause to the experiment result? Why?

Appendix: Attach Measurement of Plasma Half-Life of Sodium Salicylate

Backgrounds

Sodium salicylate turns into salicylic acid that can react with ferric chloride then form a purple complex in acidic solutions. This complex illustrates an maximum absorbance at 510 nm, which is in proportion to its concentration in Vis-UV spectrum. Measure the optical density of samples by comparing their absorbance with that of the standard, and calculate the half-life of sodium salicylate.

Materials

Same as experiment 3.

Methods

1. Weigh a rabbit and collect 2 ml of blood from its heart with a 0.5% heparin pre-moistened syringe as the standard, then inject the rabbit with 150 mg/kg of sodium salicylate solution by the ear vein.

2. Collect 2 ml of blood from rabbit's heart at 5 minutes and 35 minutes after the injection respectively.

3. Put plasma samples into 3 individual centrifuge tubes that contain 7 ml of 10% trichloroacetic acid, then centrifuge them at 1500 rpm for 5 minutes to precipitate plasma proteins.

4. Accurately draw 6 ml of supernatant from each centrifuge tubes, then put them into the test tube. Add 0.6 ml (about 12 drops) of 10% ferric chloride solution to each tube then shake well to develop colour.

5. Take the standard as control, then record the optical density (as x_1, x_2) of two supernatants at 510 nm using 1cm cuvette.

6. Calculate the half-life ($t_{1/2}$) according to the following formula:

$$t_{1/2} = \frac{0.301t}{\log x_1 - \log x_2}$$

x_1, x_2 are the optical densities of the two blood concentrations after the drug, t is the time between two blood collections.

Homework

1. Will the speed of administration and blood collection time affect the experimental results? Why?

2. How does causing drug leakage affect the experimental results? Why?

案例三　水杨酸钠药代动力学参数的测定

知识要求

1.掌握药代动力学各参数的意义，计算方法；家兔血液样本采集、处理方法。

2.熟悉水杨酸钠的药代学过程。

能力要求

1.掌握家兔血样的采集及血浆制备。

2.掌握药物的药代动力学测定方法，进行相关实验设计。

3.根据药时曲线正确计算各药代动力学参数，理解其含义。

【**实验目的**】

掌握药物血浆半衰期、表观分布容积和清除率药代动力学参数测定的意义极其测定方法。

【**实验原理**】

1.药代动力学是研究机体对药物的处置过程，通常用数学模型、药物动力学参数来表示，是新药成药性评价的关键和主要内容。通过监测药代动力学过程，可预测药物疗效和毒性、指导临床给药方案、为合理用药提供指导，实现给药方案个体化。

多数药物在体内按照一级动力学过程消除，静脉注射药物后，血浆药物浓度对数值和时间之间的关系为：

$$\lg C_t = \lg C_0 - \frac{k}{2.303}\,t \qquad (式3\text{-}3\text{-}1)$$

因此，半衰期 $t_{1/2} = 0.693/k$［单位：小时（h）或分钟（min）］　（式3-3-2）

如果按照给药后各时间点测出相应血浆药物浓度，再根据各点的分布趋势做适当直线，计算出直线斜率（s）。

由公式计算消除速率常数 $k = -2.303 \times s$ 　（式3-3-3）

根据公式3-3-2可求出 $t_{1/2}$。

表观分布容积 V_d 按照全部药量在体内分布均匀，达到血浆初始药物浓度时 C_0 所需的容积来计算。

$$V_d = \frac{静脉注射入体内药量(mg/kg)}{C_0} \quad （ml/kg 或 L/kg） \qquad (式3\text{-}3\text{-}4)$$

清除率（CL）指单位时间内机体把其中含有的药物全部加以清除的毫升数。

$$CL = \frac{0.693}{t_{1/2}} \times V_d \quad (\frac{ml}{min}/kg) \qquad (式3-3-5)$$

2.水杨酸钠浓度测定原理：在酸性环境下，水杨酸与三氯化铁形成紫色络合物，在波长520nm下的光密度值与络合物浓度成正比。

【实验材料】

1.**动物**　家兔2.5 kg，性别不限。

2.**药品**　10%水杨酸钠、0.06%水杨酸钠标准液、10%三氯醋酸、10%三氯化铁、0.5%肝素、生理盐水，二甲苯。

3.**其他材料**　兔固定箱、肝素化试管、10 ml离心管、5 ml和1 ml加样枪及枪头、5 ml注射器、6号针头、分光光度计、离心机、涡旋混匀器、手术刀片、记号笔、干棉球、一次性手套、烧杯。

【实验方法与步骤】

1.**取血**　采用肝素化试管取血。家兔称重，置入兔箱，拔去双侧耳缘静脉上的被毛。用二甲苯刺激一侧耳缘静脉，待血管扩张后，切开静脉，取3ml血液于"对照"管中，摇匀试管内血液，防止凝血。兔耳用干棉球压迫止血。

2.**给药及取血**　沿对侧耳缘静脉缓慢注射10%水杨酸钠150 mg/kg，于注射后1，3，5，10，15，20，30，45，60分钟分别通过耳缘静脉取血3 ml于不同的试管中并摇匀，静置分离血浆。

3.**测试血中水杨酸钠含量**　取离心管，分别标注为"对照"、"标准"及各时间点检测管，按下表加入样品及试剂；各管用涡旋混匀器充分混匀，以2000转/分的转速，离心10分钟。各管取上清液3 ml加入另一套干净试管中，再分别加入10%三氯化铁0.3 ml，混匀显色，利用分光光度计测定520 nm的OD值。将结果填入表3-3-1。

4.**计算药代参数**　根据OD值对应的药物浓度，以时间为横坐标，对数药物浓度为纵坐标作曲线，得到药-时曲线，根据原理中的公式（3-3-2）~（3-3-5）计算各药代参数。求C_0时，可将时量关系向纵轴方向延伸，与纵轴交点数值的反对数为C_0。

【注意事项】

1.静脉给药不能外漏，保证给药量准确。

2.给药与取血不能用同一侧兔耳。

3.取血时间尽量控制在1分钟内，取血部位也可改为颈动脉插管取血。

4.准确记录每次取血时间。

5.水杨酸钠浓度与OD值的关系可以制作标准曲线回归方程来计算，计算结果更为精确。

表 3-3-1　血样中水杨酸钠测定结果

试管号	10% 三氯醋酸 （ml）	血浆 （ml）	0.06% 水杨酸钠 （ml）	生理盐水 （ml）	OD （520 nm）
对照	4	1	0	1	
标准	4	1	1	0	
1 分钟	4	1	0	1	
3 分钟	4	1	0	1	
5 分钟	4	1	0	1	
10 分钟	4	1	0	1	
15 分钟	4	1	0	1	
20 分钟	4	1	0	1	
30 分钟	4	1	0	1	
45 分钟	4	1	0	1	
60 分钟	4	1	0	1	

附：水杨酸钠血浆浓度半衰期快速测定方法

【实验原理】

水杨酸钠在酸性环境中生成为水杨酸，水杨酸与三氯化铁反应生成一种紫色络合物。在紫外-可见光分析中，该络合物可在510nm产生吸收峰，此时光密度值与浓度成正比。根据紫色络合物的颜色进行比色，可得光密度值，将光密度值代入公式计算得半衰期。

【实验材料】

同案例三。

【实验方法】

1.取一只兔，称体重，用经0.5％肝素提前湿润过的注射器从兔心取血2 ml（作对照血样），然后从耳缘静脉注入10％水杨酸钠溶液150 mg/kg。

2.注射药物后5分钟和35分钟分别从心脏取血2 ml。

3.将上述三次抽的血浆分别放入三支预先装有7 ml 10％三氯醋酸的离心管离心（1500转/分）5分钟，使血浆蛋白沉淀。

4.准确吸取上清液各6 ml 分别置入试管内，每管加10％三氯化铁溶液0.6 ml（或12滴）摇匀后即可显色。

5.以给药前的血样为对照，在分光光度计上，设定波长510 nm，采用1 cm 光径比色皿进行比色，测定给药后两管上清液的光密度（x_1，x_2）。

6.根据下列公式求半衰期$t_{1/2}$。

$$t_{1/2} = \frac{0.301t}{\log x_1 - \log x_2}$$

式中，x_1，x_2为给药后两次血浆浓度的光密度值，t为两次取血间隔时间。

【思考题】

1.给药速度和取血时间会不会影响实验结果？为什么？

2.造成药物外漏对实验结果有何影响？为什么？

Experiment 4　Detection of *Mdr*1, an Anti–Tumour Drug Resistance Gene, by RT–PCR

Knowledge

1. Be proficient in RT-PCR experiment setting and operation process.
2. Be familiar with the mechanism of RT-PCR and how to design PCR primers.
3. Understand the mechanism of drug resistance of tumour cells, and how drug resistance gene works in this process.

Skill

1. Be proficient in the entire process of RT-PCR, including primer designing, parameter setting, gene amplification and identification.
2. Understand how to apply this method in designing experiment and measuring the level of target genes.

Objective

Detect, amplify and compare the *Mdr*1 gene in both normal and hepatic cancer cells with RT-PCR. This result would indicate the up-regulation of *Mdr*1 gene in malignant hepatic tumour cells as a significant cause of drug resistance.

Background

Malignant hepatic tumours are common cancers in China, including hepatocellular carcinoma (HCC), intrahepatic cholangiocarcinoma (ICC), and hepatocellular carcinoma-intrahepatic cholangiocarcinoma (HCC-ICC). The mortality of liver malignant tumours is relatively high due to lack of effective treatments. Liver cancers develop rapidly, whereas it's hard to diagnose them in the early stage as they have no typical clinical symptoms. Currently, surgery is the preferred treatment for liver cancers, however it's difficult to remove all tumour cells and it often has a poor prognosis. Therefore, chemotherapy plays an important role in hepatic cancer treatment, but liver malignant tumours are usually insensitive to chemotherapy drugs, and chemotherapy resistance is common, which affects the prognosis of patients.

5-Fu and its derivatives, platinum (cisplatin, oxaliplatin, etc.) and anthracyclines (doxorubicin, etc.) are commonly used chemotherapy drugs in treating liver cancer, especially the combined therapy of oxaliplatin, 5-Fu and doxorubicin to treat advanced primary liver cancer with reliable efficacy and good tolerability, however it's still limited by drug resistance.

Clinical practice illustrates that liver cancer cells are less sensitive to chemotherapy drugs than other cancers because of drug resistance. Cancer drug resistances include pan drug resistant (PDR) and multi-drug resistance (MDR), whereas MDR plays a major role in tumour defencing against chemo drugs. MDR is defined as a type of drug resistance to similar drugs after tumour cells were treated with a certain chemo-therapeutic drug. It affects drugs with similar structures and mechanisms. *Mdr*1 gene-mediate MDR is one of the complex cause of MDR.

Multi-drug resistance gene 1 (*Mdr*1) is a member of the ATP-binding cassette carrier super-family, which encodes a series of P-gp protein that can pump some intracellular anti-tumour drugs out of the cell. It can also redistribute the anti-tumour drugs in cancer cell to inhibit their efficacy. Hence, the high expression of P-gp is a main cause of MDR in tumour cells.

RT-PCR (reverse transcription-polymerase chain reaction) is commonly used in detecting *Mdr*1 genes. Its mechanism is described as follows: firstly, extract total RNA from tissues or cells, then employ the mRNA as reverse transcript templates to synthesise cDNA with Oligo (dT) or random primers. Secondly, PCR amplify the cDNA to obtain target genes or detect gene expressions. The RT-PCR method has strong specificity and high sensitivity, therefore it has been widely used in cancer diagnosis, and gradually developed.

Materials

1. Equipments: PCR machine, low-speed centrifuge, nucleic acid electrophoresis instrument, gel imaging analysis system, pipette, pipette tips, Eppendorf centrifuge tube, etc.

2. Cells: hepatic cancer cells, normal liver cells.

3. Drugs: Trizol reagent, cDNA reverse transcription kit, SYBR Green PCR Master Mix (2 ×) kit, sterile distilled water, agarose, primer, TBE buffer, DNA loading buffer, ethidium bromide, etc.

Methods

1. RNA Extraction

Extract 1 μg of total RNA from cells by Trizol method.

2. cDNA Preparation

Prepare 1-2 μg of cDNA according to the instruction of the kit. PCR-amplify the cDNA.

3. Primer Design and Synthesis

Design primers to amplify *Mdr*1 gene of 154bp, the forward primer is: 5'-CATTGGCGA-GCCTGGTAG-3', the reverse primer is 5'-TCGTAGGAGTGTCCGTGGAT-3'.

4. Reaction

The total reaction system is of 20μl volume, including 1.5μl of cDNA template, 0.2μl each of both primers, 10μl of SYBR Green Mix, and 8.1μl of ddH$_2$O.

5. Reaction Parameters

94℃ 30 s - 95℃ 10 s -60℃ 30 s for 33 cycles, then 95℃ 15 s, 60℃ 60 s, 95℃ 15 s in the final cycle.

6. Configure 0.8% Agarose Gel Solution

Put 0.4 g of agarose into a 250ml conical flask, add 50ml TBE buffer, then put the flask in a microwave oven (or on an electric stove) and heat it until the agarose is completely melted, then take it out and shake it well.

7. Pouring Agarose Gel

Insert the sample comb into the gel tank, and add ethidium bromide (EB solution) into the agarose gel solution that cooled to 50-60°C and dilute it into 0.5μg/ml, gently shake it well and carefully pour the agarose gel into the glue tank to form a flat glue layer. Pull out the comb after the glue is completely solidified.

8. Identification of PCR product

Mix the PCR product with the DNA loading buffer and add it to the loading well.Identify PCR amplification products via agarose gel electrophoresis.

9. Electrophoresis

For 30 minutes at 100 V, then observe and photo the result under UV light.

Notes

1. Follow the instruction when extract RNA and prepare cDNA.
2. Always wear gloves to avoid toxic reagent contaminations.
3. Avoid bubbles when pouring the gel.

Homework

1. Are there other methods to detect the *Mdr*1 gene?
2. What is the significance of drug resistance genetic testing to combat the precise use of anti-tumor drugs?

案例四　抗肿瘤药物精准用药——以耐药基因 *Mdr*1 检测为例（RT–PCR 法）

知识要求

1. 掌握RT-PCR实验参数设定及具体的实验操作过程。

2. 熟悉RT-PCR实验方法的原理及引物设计方法。

3. 理解分子靶向抗肿瘤药物精准诊断原理。

能力要求

1. 掌握RT-PCR方法从引物设计、参数设定、基因扩增到鉴定整个过程的操作。

2. 掌握该方法设计实验，检测耐药基因进行精准诊断的基本操作。

3. 掌握药物的药代动力学测定方法，进行相关实验设计。

【实验目的】

采用RT-PCR法检测扩增正常细胞和肝癌细胞中的*Mdr*1基因，对比说明肝癌细胞中*Mdr*1基因与抗肿瘤药物耐受的相关性情况。

【实验原理】

肝脏恶性肿瘤是我国常见的恶性肿瘤之一，主要包含肝细胞肝癌（HCC）、肝内胆管细胞癌（ICC）、肝细胞癌-肝内胆管癌（HCC-ICC）。肝脏恶性肿瘤的发病率和死亡率均处于较高水平，且导致死亡率高的直接原因之一是目前尚缺乏有效的治疗手段。肝恶性肿瘤具有起病隐匿、入侵快、死亡率高的特点，同时缺乏典型临床症状，手术是目前首选的治疗方案，但由于其发现时多处于晚期，难以根治性切除，预后差。所以化疗是其重要的治疗手段，但肝恶性肿瘤对化疗药物通常不敏感，且易出现化疗耐药性，影响患者预后。

通常用于肝癌治疗的化学治疗药物包括5-Fu及其衍生物（铂类，奥沙利铂）和蒽环霉素；其中奥沙利铂、5-Fu和多柔比星的联合用药被广泛用于治疗晚期原发性肝癌，并且疗效可靠，耐受性好，但其化学抗性仍然是限制其应用的一个持久难题。

临床实践表明肝癌细胞对化学治疗药物的敏感性低于许多其他癌症，其主要原因是出现了耐药现象。肿瘤耐药包括原药耐药及多药耐药（MDR），而MDR在肿瘤细胞防御化疗药物攻击中起主要作用。MDR是指肿瘤细胞接触某种化疗药物后产生抗性，不仅只针对与这种药物结构类似的药物，对其他不同化学结构和作用机制的药物同样产生抗性。MDR产生的机制较为复杂，而MDR1介导的耐药机制则是其中一种较为经典的作用机制。

MDR1是ATP结合盒载体超家族成员之一，其基因编码的蛋白产物P-gp具有能量依赖性药泵功能，可将细胞内多种抗肿瘤药物泵出细胞外，还可使抗肿瘤药物在细胞内再分布，从而使抗肿瘤药物无法有效杀灭肿瘤细胞，并产生耐药性。P-gp高表达是肿瘤细胞MDR的主要原因。

*Mdr*1基因的检测多用RT-PCR法，即反转录-聚合酶链反应。其原理是：提取组织或细胞中的总RNA，以其中的mRNA作为模板，采用Oligo（dT）或随机引物通过反转录酶反转录成cDNA。再以cDNA为模板进行PCR扩增，从而获得目的基因或检测基因表达。RT-PCR法具有特异性强，灵敏度高的优点，因而在检测诊断领域得到广泛应用，并逐步被发展和完善。

【实验材料】

1.仪器　PCR仪，台式低速离心机，核酸电泳仪，凝胶成像分析仪，移液器，Tip头（移液器替换头），Eppendorf离心管等。

2.细胞　肝癌细胞、正常细胞。

3.药品　Trizol试剂、cDNA反转录试剂盒、SYBR Green PCR Master Mix（2×）试剂盒、引物、无菌蒸馏水、琼脂糖、TBE缓冲液、核酸上样缓冲液、溴化乙啶等。

【实验方法】

1.RNA的提取　Trizol法提取细胞总RNA，得到1μg总RNA。

2. cDNA制备　根据反转录试剂盒使用说明制备cDNA1~2μg。以cDNA为模板，按照SYBR Green PCR Master Mix（2×）试剂盒说明进行PCR扩增。

3.引物设计与合成　设计引物用于扩增Mdr1基因154bp。Mdr1正向引物：5'-CATTGGCGAGCCTGGTAG-3'，反向引物：5'-TCGTAGGAGTGTCCGTGGAT-3'。

4.反应体系　共20μl：cDNA模板1.5μl，上下游引物各0.2μl，SYBR Green Mix试剂10μl，ddH$_2$O 8.1μl。

5.反应条件设定　反应条件：设定扩增参数为94℃ 30秒，95℃ 10秒，60℃ 30秒共33个循环，最后一个循环的扩增参数为95℃ 15秒，60℃ 60秒，95℃ 15秒。

6.配置0.8%琼脂糖凝胶液　称取0.4 g琼脂糖，置于250 ml锥形瓶中，加入50 ml TBE缓冲液，放入微波炉里（或电炉上）加热至琼脂糖全部溶解，取出摇匀。

7.灌制琼脂糖凝胶　将胶槽插上样品梳子，向冷却至50~60℃的琼脂糖凝胶液中加入溴化乙啶（EB溶液），使其终浓度为0.5μg/ml，轻轻摇匀，将琼脂糖凝胶液小心地倒入胶槽内，使胶液形成均匀的胶层。待胶完全凝固后拨出梳子。

8.鉴定PCR扩增产物　将PCR产物混合上样缓冲液后加入上样孔，通过琼脂糖凝胶电泳法鉴定PCR扩增产物。

9.电泳　将凝胶放入电泳仪设定电压为100 V，电泳30分钟；将凝胶置于凝胶成像分析仪中并打开紫外模式，于紫外灯下观察结果并照相记录。

【注意事项】

1.按照试剂盒操作说明提取RNA，制备cDNA。

2.实验过程应佩戴手套，避免有毒试剂沾染皮肤。

3.灌制凝胶的时候注意不要产生气泡。

【思考题】

1.Mdr1基因的其他检测方法有哪些？

2.耐药基因检测对抗肿瘤药物精准使用有什么重要意义？

第四篇
临床药理学实习

Chapter 4
Clinical Pharmacology Practice

I. Pharmacy Services

Pharmacy services refer to services that ensure the safety of patients' medication optimise the treatment effect and save costs, provided by pharmacy professionals (pharmacist), aiming at detecting and solving medication-related problems. Pharmacy services involve outpatient clinics, hospitalizations, and home pharmacies, including but not limited to pharmacy clinics, prescription review, medication reorganization, medication consultation, medication education, pharmacy ward rounds, medication monitoring, home pharmacy services, etc.

1. Contents of Pharmacy Service

1.1 Outpatient pharmacy services: pharmacy clinics, prescription review, drug reorganization, medication consultation, medication education, etc.

1.2 Inpatient pharmacy services: pharmacy ward rounds, medication monitoring, prescription review, medication reorganization, medication consultation, medication education, etc.

1.3 Home pharmacy services: home pharmacy services, medication reformation, medication consultation, medication education, etc.

2. Pharmacy Service Process

The process of pharmacy service includes collecting information, information analysing and evaluating, making plans, executing plans, and following up.

2.1 The content of information collection includes basic patient information (age, gender, address, medical insurance, etc.), health information (personal history, family history, reproductive history, past medical history, current medical history, living habits, etc.), medication information (medication history, medications, etc.) Adverse reaction history, immunisation history, etc., demand information (drug treatment, health status, pharmacist services), etc. Collected information includes standardised information collection and individualised information collection.

（1）Standardised information collection means pharmacists and patients obtain patient information through various methods such as consulting hospital's electronic medical record system before meeting, so as to provide a basis for the subsequent implementation of standardised pharmaceutical services and improve the efficiency of pharmaceutical services.

（2）Individualized information collection means pharmacists conduct pharmacy consultations during face-to-face interviews with patients, and supply individualized information based on differences in disease condition, health literacy, communication skill, and willingness to communicate.

2.2 Pharmaceutical service analysis and evaluation refers to the comprehensive evaluation and analysis of collected information, and the discovery of patients' existing and potential drug treatment-related problems. Pharmacists evaluate the insufficiency of drug treatment plans, excessive drug treatment, ineffective drug treatments, insufficient drug dosage, adverse drug events, excessive drug dosage, and poor compliance, in terms of indications, effectiveness, safety, and compliance. Pharmacists systematically and comprehensively analyse and evaluate medication-related issues for patients, sort them according to their urgency and importance, and intervene 3 to 5 medication-related issues each time, facilitating the implementation of subsequent intervention plans.

（1）Excessive drug treatment includes medication without indications, excessive combination therapy, unnecessary drug treatment, and using drugs to treat adverse reactions caused by other drugs.

（2）Insufficient drug treatment program includes conditions that need initiating new drugs to treat diseases, preventive medications to reduce the risk of new diseases, increasing the dosage to obtain synergistic or additional therapeutic effects.

（3）Ineffective drug therapy includes the patient's resistance to drugs, improper drug formulation or route of administration, and ineffective drug therapy.

（4）Insufficient drug dosage includes too low drug doses, too long medication intervals, drug interactions that weaken the dosage, and the too short treatment period.

（5）Adverse drug events include adverse reactions that are not related to drug dosage, requirements of safer drugs due to risk factors, adverse reactions caused by drug interactions but not related to dosage, too rapid adjustments of the medication regimen, drug-related allergy reactions, patient's contraindications, and the misuse or improper use of dosage forms.

（6）Excessive drug doses include too high single doses, too short medication intervals, too long medication duration, medication-related toxic reactions due to drug interactions, and too-fast administration.

（7）Poor compliance includes patients who do not fully understand medication instructions, patients that are subjectively unwilling to take drugs, patients who forget taking medications, patients that refuse taking drug due to the cost, patients who cannot take or use medications by themselves, and patients that cannot obtain drugs by themselves.

2.3. Based on the result of the analysis and evaluation, pharmacists shall formulate a clear, quantifiable, achievable intervention plan that can be accurately understood by the patient, and a specific completion timetable shall be given.

2.4. According to the intervention plan, the pharmacist can advise the prescribing physician to change the patient's treatment plan (such as adding new treatment drugs, stopping treatment, increasing the dose, reducing the dose, etc.).

2.5. Pharmacists conduct follow-ups based on the patient's diseases and medication conditions, with the purpose of assessing the implementation of the intervention plan, meeting the standards of disease monitoring indicators, adjusting the intervention plan if necessary, and tracking the effectiveness of the implementation of pharmaceutical services.

II. Pharmacy Clinic

Pharmacy clinic refers to a series of professional services that provided by pharmacists with professional and technical advantages in pharmacy to patients, such as medication evaluation, medication adjustment, drug plan, medication education, follow-up guidance, etc., in medical institutions.

1. Form

1.1 Independent Pharmacist Pharmacy Clinic: such as specialist outpatient clinics and comprehensive outpatient clinics.

1.2 Pharmacist participation in outpatient clinics: including physician-pharmacist cooperative outpatient clinics and multidisciplinary cooperative outpatient clinics.

2. The Service Process

Pharmacy clinic serve patients who have questions about medication, focusing on the following patients:

2.1 Patients that suffer from one or more chronic diseases and receive treatment of multiple systems, including patients with chronic kidney diseases, hypertension, diabetes, hyperlipidemia, coronary heart disease, stroke and other diseases.

2.2 Patients who take 5 or more drugs at the same time.

2.3 Patients who are taking special drugs, such as alerted drugs, glucocorticoids, drugs with special dosage forms, drugs with special administration time, etc.

2.4 Special population: the elderly, children, pregnant and lactating women, liver and kidney dysfunction patients, etc.

2.5 Patients that suspected of having adverse drug reactions.

2.6 Patients who need pharmacists to interpret the therapeutic drug monitoring report, including blood drug concentration and drug genetic testing.

3. Contents of Pharmacy Outpatient Clinic

Pharmacy outpatient clinic contains the collection of patient information, drug treatment evaluation, medication plan adjustment, formulation of drug treatment-related action plans, patient education and follow-up.

3.1 Collection of Patient Information: including their basic information, personal history, living habits, patient concerns, special needs, medical history, past and current medication history, history of adverse drug reaction, drug compliance, immunization history, auxiliary examination results, etc.

3.2 Evaluation of Drug Treatment: the visiting pharmacist should analyse the indications, effectiveness, safety, and compliance. The medication analysis is based on evidence but not limited to comprehensive analysis. Focus on the treatment needs of patients, and provide specific recommendations based on the patient's individual conditions, diseases, and medications used.

3.3 Adjustment of Medication Plan: pharmacists can adjust the treatment plan by means of agreement on prescriptions and communication with relevant physicians.

3.4 Formulate Action Plans Related to Drug Treatments: including medication recommendations, lifestyle adjustments, and referrals.

3.5 Patient Education: provide guidance on drug's indications, usage and dosage, precautions, adverse reactions and lifestyle adjustments, to verify the patient's understanding and acceptance of the pharmacist's recommendations.

3.6 Follow-Up: set a follow-up plan based on the patient's condition. Contents of the follow-up include the evaluation of drug treatment goals, the occurrence of new treatment-related problems, if the drug adverse reaction occurs, if the medication compliance is good, and inspect the follow-up result.

III. Prescription Review

Prescription review refers to the review of the legality, standardisation, and suitability of prescriptions issued by doctors for patients in diagnosis and treatment activities in accordance with relevant laws and regulations, rules and regulations, and decide whether to dispense the drug, based on professional knowledge and skills.

1.Objects of Prescription Review

It Contains out patient and emergency prescriptions and inpatient orders issued by physicians in the institution or partner units. The form of prescriptions includes: prescriptions in paper, electronic prescriptions, and ward medication orders.

2. Forms of Prescription Review

2.1 Manual Review: the pharmacist reviews the legality, standardisation, and suitability of the prescription, one by one.

2.2 System-Assisted Prescription Review: the medical institution should form an information system with software for rational drug use. These softwares may conduct preliminary prescription reviews. Those prescriptions that are rejected by the software should be manually reviewed by the pharmacist.

3. The Basis for Prescription Review

It includes drug instructions, national drug management related laws and regulatory documents, national formulary, clinical diagnosis and treatment specifications and guidelines issued by the national health authority, clinical pathways, etc.

4. The Process of Prescription Review

4.1 Receive prescriptions to be reviewed, and review the prescriptions in terms of legality, standardisation, and suitability.

4.2 If the prescription is judged to be a reasonable prescription after the review, the pharmacist should sign the prescription, then the prescription will enter the charging and dispensing stage after the review.

4.3 If the prescription is determined to unreasonable after the review, pharmacist will contact the prescribing physician to modify or re-issue the prescription. Then, the re-issued prescription by the prescribing physician will be reviewed again. If the physician does not agree to modify or re-issue the prescription, the pharmacist shall keep a record, and refuse the prescription if it has serious unreasonable medication errors then report it to the medical department. Reasonable prescriptions should be dispensed, and the pharmacist should verify the medicine and guide patients in terms of administration routes and time, dosage, precautions, etc. For prescriptions that can not be accurately judged, the pharmacist should communicate with the prescribing physician, seek support from superior pharmacists and physicians if necessary. Fig. 4.3.1 illustrates the process of the work of prescription review pharmacist.

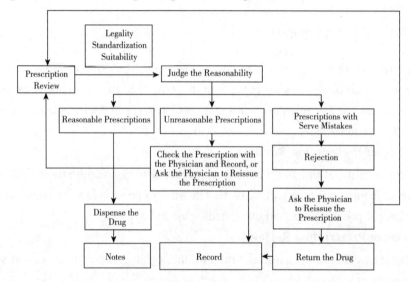

Figure 4.3.1. The Process of Prescription Review

IV. Medication Consultation

Medication consultation refers to the process in which pharmacists provide medication information, promote knowledge of rational drug use and to exchange medication-related issues, to patients, their families, medical staff, and the public.

1. Objects of Medication Consultation Services

These include patients, their families, medical staff, and the public.

2. Route of Medication Consultation

It contains face-to-face consultation, telephone consultation and Internet consultation.

3. Medication Consultation

It may includes the name of the drug, usage and dosage, efficacy, medication precautions, drug interactions, storage methods, identification treatment of adverse drug reactions, special formulation guidance, patient medication education and disease prevention, etc.

4. The Process of Medication Consultation

It includes receiving consultants, inquiring their need, collecting medication history and related medical history, analysing and evaluating, and answering questions from consultants in time. During the consultation, pharmacists should record relevant information, including name, gender and date of birth of the consultant, drug name, consultation questions, answer content, and reference basis, etc.

V. Medication Reorganization

Medication reorganisation refers to the process of comparing whether all the medications being used by the patient are consistent with the order. Its detailed definition includes that the pharmacist communicates or reviews with the patient to understand whether the overall medication situation before and after the medical handover is consistent at each stage of the treatment, such as admission, transfer or discharge. And make adjustments to unsuitable medications to prevent adverse drug events and ensure the safety of patients' medication.

1. The Implementation Process of Reorganization

Drug reorganization should be carried out through the entire medical process, especially when the medical team changes, including admission, transfer or discharge. For all adjustments in drugs, fully communicate with the physician, and collect medication history through interviews with patients or their families and access to patients' past medical records and prescription information. The past medication history should include name, dosage form and specification, usage and dosage, start and stop of the medicine currently used and the medicines closely related to the disease, such as the compliance to prescription drugs, over-the-counter medicines, Chinese patent drugs/Chinese herbal medicines and vaccines, and health care products, etc. Information about the history of drug and food allergies should also be collected. The pharmacist should establish a medication reorganization record based on the past medication history.

2. Contents That Should Be Focused on During the Drug Reorganization

2.1 Check the indication and whether there are repeated medications.

2.2 Check whether the administrate route and dosage are correct.

2.3 Pay attention to drugs with special dosage forms/devices and whether the route of administration is appropriate.

2.4 Pay attention to the drugs that need to be adjusted according to liver and kidney functions, and adjust the dosage if necessary.

2.5 Pay attention to drugs with potential interactions and possible adverse reactions, and adjust the treatment plan if necessary.

2.6 Pay attention to symptom-relieving drugs, which are the focus of reorganization, and clarify whether these drugs can be long-term used.

2.7 Pay attention to special populations, such as the elderly, children, pregnant and lactating women, patients with liver and kidney dysfunctions, mental illness patients, etc. Comprehensively consider the safety, effectiveness, suitability and compliance of these patients' medication.

2.8 Check whether certain drugs need to be temporarily stopped before the planned inspection or medical operation, and evaluate whether to continue the drug after the operation.

2.9 Pay attention to whether intravenous drugs and drugs with a clear course of treatment can continue to be used.

VI. Medication Education

Medication education refers to the guidance of rational use of medicines and popularise knowledge of rational use of medicines to patients. The purpose of this section is to enhance patients' understand of medication, in order to prevent adverse drug reactions, improve patient compliance, and reduce the incidence of medication errors.

1. Steps of Medication Education

1.1 Introduce yourself to the patient and explain the purpose and expected time of this education.

1.2 Collect the patient's disease history, medication history, education level and other information to determine the method of medication education, oral or written, based on preliminary communication, and fully consider the patient's conditions, such as vision, hearing, language barriers, etc.

1.3 Assess the patient's understanding and expectation of their health problems and medications, their ability to use medications correctly, and their attitude towards treatment.

1.4 Assess the patient's understand of the purpose of medication, administration routes, dosage, medication course, precautions, common adverse reactions, etc. Set individualised medication educational programs according to the patient's understand.

1.5 Adopt one or more education methods for individual patients for medication education, in order to ensure the patient understands the importance of medication and use the drug correctly.

1.6 Before the end of the education, the patient's knowledge of medication use should be verified. Ask the patient to repeat the key content of medication education, adjust the medication education method according to patient's receiving effect, and conduct medication education again until the patient fully grasps it.

1.7 Truthfully record the medication education record.

2. Contents of Medication Education

2.1 The generic name, trade name, or other commonly used names of the drug or medical device, as well as the drug's classification, usage and expected effects.

2.2 Estimated time of the drug taking effect and the response action if it does not take effect.

2.3 Dosage form, route of administration, dosage, medication time and the course of the treatment.

2.4 The specific dosage form, special device, and special preparation method of the drug, which can be adjusted due to the patient's lifestyle or living environment.

2.5 Symptoms, signs and test indicators that should be monitored during the medication. Explain possible interferences to clinical tests and changes in the colour of excrement by the drug.

2.6 Common and serious adverse reactions that may occur, preventive measures that can be taken, and emergency measures to be taken after adverse reactions. Possible results in case of medication errors, such as missed dosing, and measures that should to be taken.

2.7 Potential drug-drug, drug-food/health products, drug-disease and drug-environment interactions or contraindications.

2.8 Appropriate storage conditions for drugs, proper disposal of expired drugs or discarded devices.

2.9 Methods to make medication records and self-monitoring, to contact the pharmacist in time.

VII. Pharmacy Ward Rounds

Pharmacy rounds refer to the process of ward rounds with clinical pharmacists as the main body to ensure the safe, reasonable and effective medication, including independent rounds of pharmacists and joint rounds of pharmacists, physicians, and nurses.

1. The Environment and Objects of Pharmacy Rounds

1.1 Clinical pharmacists should conduct pharmacy rounds in selected clinical departments.

1.2 Clinical pharmacists should conduct pharmacy rounds for patients who refer for pharmacy consultation.

1.3 The place for routine pharmacy rounds should be beside the bedside.

2. Preparation for the Ward Rounds

2.1 Clarify the number of patients for pharmacy rounds and expected time for them.

2.2 Obtain and be familiar with basic situations of the patient, especially patients that are critically ill, severely ill, in complicated condition and newly admitted patients, including but not limited to the patient's name, gender, age, vital signs, current medical history, underlying diseases, disease history, medication history, allergy history, family history, personal history, marriage and childbirth history, hospital admission diagnosis, auxiliary examination results, treatment plan, disease progression, etc.

2.3 When familiarise with the patient's information, make records for the part that has questions or focus on.

2.4 Reorganise the drug used outside the hospital for newly admitted patients, sort out the initial treatment plan for the patient, and conduct key monitoring drugs, such as antibacterial drugs, glucocorticoids, anti-tumour drugs and some key drugs of various specialties.

2.5 Analyse the rationality of the initial treatment plan in effectiveness, safety, economy, and suitability of the drug, then record and intervene in unreasonable medical orders.

（1）The analysis of drug effectiveness should include but not be limited to drug indications, usage and dosage, route of administration and course of treatment, etc.

（2）Drug safety analysis includes the prevention and treatment of adverse drug reactions, evaluation of drug interactions, etc.

（3）Economic analysis of medication use contains medical insurance and patient affordability, etc.

（4）The drug suitability analysis includes skin test results, drug specifications and repeated drug use, etc.

2.6 The analysis of orders for patients in hospital should consider their disease progression, auxiliary test results and treatment plan adjustments, etc., especially the diagnosis revision that may affect medication, the update of laboratory examination results (such as liver and kidney function changes, etc.), the change of combined medication, and changes of doctor's important orders, etc. Through the analysis of rational drug use, extract the ideas and contents of pharmacy rounds such as the content of pharmacy consultation and main points of patient education.

2.7 Contents of the round record form for newly admitted patients should include the basic condition of the patient, the patient's diagnosis, laboratory test results, out-of-hospital medical order reorganization, initial treatment plan, medication effectiveness, safety, economy and suitability analysis, irrational medication intervention, pharmacy consultation content, compliance evaluation, patient education, questions and patient feedback, etc. Content of the patient rounds record form in the hospital should include but not be limited to basic situations of the patient, patient diagnosis, revised diagnosis, update of laboratory examination results, adjustment of treatment plan, analysis of the effectiveness, safety, economy and suitability of the adjusted plan, irrational medication intervention, pharmacy consultation content, patient education, questions and patient feedback, etc.

3. Process of the Ward Round

3.1 During the initial round of patients, a simple self-introduction should be made to inform the patient of the identity of clinical pharmacists and the pharmaceutical service during the stay. Informing patients that the main purpose of pharmacy rounds is to provide precautions related to the medication and to promote the rational use of drugs.

3.2 Main contents of pharmacy consultation include all disease and drug-related information in the entire diagnosis and treatment process of the patient, to evaluate benefits and risks of the patient's drug treatment and obtain the treatment needs of the patient, and provides basic information and objective evidence for the implementation of pharmaceutical care.

3.3 Focus on the patient's medication, verify if the patient is taking the medication as required, reactions after the medication, if there is any discomfort, hobby, lifestyle and other information, in order to carry out targeted medication education, guide the patient to use the drug correctly and develop a pharmaceutical care plan.

3.4 For newly admitted patients, pharmacists should actively communicate with patients or their family members, and ask them about the treatment purpose, previous diseases and treatment history, history of medication and food allergies, adverse drug reactions, and other basic information. As for the previous medication, name of the drug, drug specifications, administration routes, dosage, course of treatment, efficacy, etc., should be inquired in detail. If the patient has drug allergy, name of the drug, allergy symptoms, signs, and outcome should all be asked.

3.5 For patients in the process of diagnosis and treatment, they should be asked about their own diseases, their understand of medications, and whether they are taking medications as required. Ask patients about the improvement in symptoms and signs after using the drug, whether they have new symptoms, and determine the efficacy of patient's current treatment. Develop a monitoring plan, including changes in patient indicators, judgment of adverse reactions, changes in dosing regimens, and whether dosing regimens need to be adjusted, etc.

3.6 Method of medication education include education by language, in written and by physical demonstration. The medication education contains universal medication education, medication education for special dosage forms, medication education for special populations, and medication education for special drugs. Specific contents of the medication education should include the name of the drug, both the trade name and the generic name, drug specifications, drug properties, reasons for medication, usage and dosage, time of medication, including fasting/meal/after meals, etc., and method of medication, such as swallowing, chewing, and so on, common adverse reactions, precautions, including drug-drug, drug-food interactions, strategies to handle missed doses, and storage methods, etc. As well as diet, lifestyle, disease-related indicators, including blood pressure, blood lipids, blood sugar, etc.,medication monitoring and follow-up visits. After the education, materials should be distributed to patients to consolidate the result of it.

3.7 According to the result of the evaluation, clinical pharmacists should sort out the patient's medication problems, search the literature, analyse the problems, offer solutions and suggestions for the problems, and communicate with the doctors, nurses and patients in time.

VIII. Medication Monitoring

Medication monitoring refers to direct, responsible, drug use-related monitoring to inpatients with professional pharmaceutical knowledge in order to improve the safety, effectiveness and economy of drug treatment.

Graded medication monitoring refers to the determination of care level by the pharmacist based on the patient's disease state, disease characteristics, and medication during the hospitalisation.

Process of Medication Monitoring

1. Medication monitoring of inpatients should be carried throughout the entire treatment, from the time the patient enters the ward for consultation, to when the patient is transferred or discharged from the hospital. If the patient is transferred to another department, the pharmacist should re-assess and monitor the patient again.

2. Determine the care to the patient, the patient's pathophysiological state, etc. Pharmacists should classify the medication monitoring services due to the medication monitoring grading standards. For patients in special specialties, such as tumour, haematology, paediatrics, etc., it can be adjusted according to above standards.

3. Pharmacists may carry out medication monitoring classification and different levels of medication monitoring referring to classification medication monitoring.They can also apply methods such as drug gene testing, therapeutic drug monitoring in drug monitoring, combined with pharmacokinetics and pharmacodynamics, to formulate individualised drug treatment plans and carry out medication monitoring on patients.

4. Establish a standardised medication monitoring record form, and truthfully record the patient's medication treatment during the hospitalisation.

5. For inappropriate treatments, pharmacists should record specific suggestions, reference basis, and feedback results from physicians and/or nurses.

IX. Home Pharmacy Service

Home pharmacy services refers to individualised, full-course, continuous pharmacy services and popularisation of health knowledge for home medications, provided by medical institutions, conducting medication evaluation and medication education, helping patients improve medication compliance, and ensuring the safe and reasonable storage and use of medications, to improve the treatment result. During this process, pharmacists can prepare medicine boxes, medicine teaching tools, such as insulin pens, inhalation preparation devices, etc., measuring instruments, such as blood glucose meters, sphygmomanometers, weight scales, peak flow meters, tapes, etc., and forms for patient management with chronic diseases according to their needs, such as peak flow rate record table, and other items.

1. Service Process

Home pharmacy service mainly targets on patients who have contracted with the family doctor service and key patients who are prone to drug-related problems.

2. Home Pharmacy Service Includes But It not Limited to the Following Contents

2.1 Medication reorganization and medication management for patients with high diagnosis times and residents with a large number of drugs, pharmacists can provide medication reorganization and management services, and suggestions, then contact the patient's attending doctor or other specialists and finally determine the patient's new treatment plan. Pharmacists should also provide comprehensive guidance and medication education to patients.

2.2 Medication consultation: when patients have questions or concerns about their medications, pharmacists may provide medication consultation services.

2.3 Medication education: for special patients and special drugs, pharmacists may provide medication education service. Special patients include: patients who have recently experienced important changes in drug therapy, such as returning home after being discharged, unconscious or unable to swallow the complete drug. Special drugs contain high-risk drugs, such as the anticoagulant, insulin, drugs with a narrow therapeutic window, and drugs with complex devices, such as inhaled preparations, etc.

2.4 Science popularisation and education: conduct popular science publicity for home patients with personalised science popularisation and education methods and easy-to-understand language to disseminate correct drug information to patients, to keep the drug use safe, effective, economical and appropriate.

2.5 Cleaning the household medicine box: pharmacists could regularly or irregularly check the validity period and properties of drugs in the patient's home, and provide guidance on the storage of drugs and the recovery of expired or spoiled medicines.

3. The General Process of Home Pharmacy Services

3.1 When provide services in primary medical institutions or the patient's home, pharmacists should wear overalls, badge, and provide services at the appointed time.

3.2 Provide pharmacy services to patients in accordance with the formulated plan.

3.3 In case of making adjustments to the patient's prescription, pharmacists should firstly communicate with the doctor, and submit the adjustment proposal in written form to the doctor for reference, then the doctor will ameliorate the prescription.

3.4 Record the content of services, such as the drug list, etc.

3.5 Discovered drug-related problems should be informed to the patient and the doctor, and recorded in the intervention record sheet.

3.6 After the service, the pharmacist should ask the client or guardian to confirm and sign the completion of the service.

3.7 If the patient needs service again, the pharmacist should arrange the next service time with the patient, and record the the next follow-up time and changes in the patient's laboratory indicators in the follow-up form.

4. References for Home Pharmacy Service

These include drug instructions, national drug management related laws and regulations and normative documents, national formulary, clinical diagnosis and treatment norms and guidelines, clinical pathways, etc. Findings during the service, and results of the communication between the pharmacist, the patient, and the physician should be recorded and kept traceable.

X. Emergency Pharmacy Service

Emergency pharmacy is a branch of pharmacy service, mainly executed by emergency pharmacists in the emergency pharmacy in hospital. The service time of emergency pharmacy is mainly after the shift and at nights. Emergency pharmacy is the cooperation between emergency and pharmacy.

1. Features of Emergency Pharmacy Services

Medical staff passively deal with emergency patients that suffer from poisoning, trauma, accidents, severe illness, transfer to hospitals, infants, young children, and elderly and weak patients. Patients in emergencies are mainly in acute illness and emotionally unstable, etc.

2. Contents of Emergency Pharmacy Services

2.1 It is necessary to prepare medicines reasonably to ensure adequate emergency medicines. A special area for emergency medicines should be set up to facilitate the dispensary of emergency medicines. Pharmacists must be familiar with the 'Emergency Pharmacy Rescue Drug List', 'Anti-Terrorism Health Emergency Drug List' and other relevant first-aid drug lists. They should also be proficient in applying the 'Inventory Warning' system and daily receive requested medicines. Emergency pharmacists should regularly check the quantity and expiry of emergency drugs to ensure that the storage is consistent with the inventory to ensure the quality of medicines.

2.2 Fully review the drug interaction, compatibility, contraindications, drug usage and dosage, and administration route. The pharmacist should immediately contact the physician and provide recommendations and intervene before the use when found unreasonable prescriptions to ensure drug safety.

2.3 Carry out medication consultation and provide accurate pharmaceutical information: for rugs that require special attention and are newly introduced, the pharmacist should carefully read the instruction and timely feedback to the physician or provide relevant information. Carefully answer questions about the medication of patients at the window, and relieve their psychological barriers.

2.4 Pay attention to allergic reactions: when review prescriptions, pharmacists should pay attention to the following information:

（1）Drugs whose instructions clearly require skin test.

（2）Patients that easily get allergy.

（3）Patients with penicillin or cephalosporin allergy history, or positive skin test history.

（4）If the dosage in the prescription is too large, communicate with the doctor.

一、药学服务

药学服务是指由药学专业技术人员（以下简称药师）为保障患者用药安全、优化患者治疗效果和节约治疗费用而进行的相关服务，旨在发现和解决与患者用药相关问题。药学服务涉及门诊、住院、居家三种场所，包括但不限于药学门诊、处方审核、药物重整、用药咨询、用药教育、药学查房、用药监护、居家药学服务等。

（一）药学服务内容

1. 门诊药学服务　包括但不限于药学门诊、处方审核、药物重整、用药咨询、用药教育等。

2. 住院药学服务　包括但不限于药学查房、用药监护、处方审核、药物重整、用药咨询、用药教育等。

3. 居家药学服务　包括但不限于居家药学服务、药物重整、用药咨询、用药教育等。

（二）药学服务流程

药学服务流程包括收集信息、分析评估、制定计划、执行计划、跟踪随访。

1. 信息收集内容包括患者基本信息（年龄、性别、住址、医保等）、健康信息（个人史、家族史、生育史、既往病史、现病史、生活习惯等）、用药信息（用药史、药物不良反应史、免疫接种史等）、需求信息（药物治疗、健康状况、药师服务）等。收集信息包括标准化信息收集和个体化信息收集。

（1）标准化信息收集是指药师与患者见面前通过查阅医院电子病历系统等各种途径获取患者信息，为后续实施规范化药学服务提供基础，提高药学服务的效率。

（2）个体化信息收集是指药师与患者进行面谈时进行药学问诊，根据患者的个体疾病差异、健康素养差异、沟通能力差异，以及沟通意愿差异等进行个体化信息补充。

2. 药学服务分析评估是指将收集到的信息进行综合评估分析，发现患者存在或潜在的药物治疗相关问题。药师从适应证、有效性、安全性、依从性4个维度展开，评估4个维度涵盖的药物治疗方案不足、药物治疗过度、无效的药物治疗、药物剂量不足、药物不良事件、药物剂量过高和用药依从性差7个方向。药师系统、全面地分析评估患者存在的药物治疗相关问题，按其紧急和重要程度进行排序，每次选择3~5个药物治疗相关问题进行干预，以利于后续干预计划的实施。

（1）药物治疗过度　包括无适应证用药、过度的联合治疗、无须药物治疗、用1种药物治疗其他药物引起的不良反应。

（2）药物治疗方案不足　包括需要启动新的药物治疗疾病、需要预防用药来降低新发疾病的风险和需要增加药物以获得协同或附加治疗效应。

（3）无效的药物治疗　包括患者对药物产生耐药、药物剂型或给药途径不当、药物治疗无效。

（4）药物剂量不足　包括药物剂量过低、用药间隔时间过长、药物相互作用减弱了有效药物剂量、药物治疗时间过短。

（5）药物不良事件　包括产生了与药物剂量无关的不良反应、由于风险因素需要选择更安全的药物、药物相互作用引起的与剂量无关的不良反应、给药方案调整过快、药物相关的过敏反应、患者存在用药禁忌证、用法用量或剂型使用不当。

（6）药物剂量过高　包括单次剂量过高、用药间隔时间太短、用药持续时间太长、因药物相互作用导致药物相关的毒性反应、给药速度过快。

（7）用药依从性差　包括患者没有充分理解用药指导或用药说明、患者主观上不愿意服药、患者忘记服药、患者认为药费过于昂贵而拒绝服药、患者不能自行服用或使用药物、患者无法获得药物。

3. 药师根据分析评估的结果，制订清晰明确、可量化、可实现、使患者能够准确理解的干预计划，并且应给出具体的完成时间。

4. 药师可按照干预计划，建议处方医师更改患者的治疗方案（如新增治疗药物、停止治疗药物、增加给药剂量、减少给药剂量等）。

5. 药师根据患者病情和用药情况，进行跟踪随访，目的是评估干预方案的实施情况和疾病监测指标的达标情况，必要时进行干预方案的调整；对实施药学服务后的成效进行跟踪。

二、药学门诊

药学门诊，是指医疗机构具有药学专业技术优势的药师对患者提供用药评估、用药调整、用药计划、用药教育、随访指导等一系列专业化服务。

（一）药学形式

1. 药师独立门诊　包含专科门诊和综合门诊。
2. 药师参与门诊　包括医师–药师联合门诊和多学科合作门诊。

（二）服务过程

药学门诊服务于任何对用药有疑问的患者，重点包括如下患者：

1. 患有1种或多种慢性病，接受多系统、多专科同时治疗的患者，例如，患有慢性肾病、高血压、糖尿病、高脂血症、冠心病、脑卒中等疾病的患者；

2. 同时服用5种及以上药物的患者；

3. 正在服用特殊药物的患者：包括高警示药品、糖皮质激素、特殊剂型药物、特殊给药时间药物等；

4. 特殊人群：老年人、儿童、妊娠期与哺乳期妇女、肝肾功能不全者等；

5. 怀疑发生药物不良反应的患者；

6. 需要药师解读治疗药物监测（如血药浓度和药物基因检测）报告的患者。

（三）药学门诊服务内容

包括收集患者信息、药物治疗评价、用药方案调整、制定药物治疗相关行动计划、患者教育和随访六个环节。

1. 收集患者信息　包括基本信息、个人史、生活习惯、患者关切的问题、特殊需求、病史、既往史和当前用药史、药物不良反应史、用药依从性、免疫接种史、辅助检查结果等。

2. 药物治疗评价　出诊药师从适应证、有效性、安全性、依从性等方面进行分析。用药分析时基于循证证据但不局限于证据进行综合分析。重点关注患者的治疗需求，结合患者个体情况、所患疾病、所用药物提出个体化建议。

3. 用药方案调整　药师可通过协议处方权、与相关医师沟通等方式进行治疗方案的调整。

4. 制定药物治疗相关行动计划　包括用药建议、生活方式调整、转诊等范畴。

5. 患者教育　对药品的适应证、用法用量、注意事项、不良反应及生活方式调整等进行指导，核实患者对药师建议的理解和接受程度。

6. 随访　根据患者情况制定随访计划，随访内容包括药物治疗目标评价、是否出现新的药物治疗相关问题、是否发生药物不良反应、用药依从性是否良好、跟踪检查结果等。

三、处方审核

处方审核，是指药学专业技术人员运用专业知识与实践技能，根据相关法律法规、规章制度与技术规范等，对医师在诊疗活动中为患者开具的处方，进行合法性、规范性和适宜性审核，并做出是否同意调配发药决定的药学技术服务。

（一）处方审核对象

包括本机构或合作单位医师开具的门急诊处方和住院医嘱，处方形式包括：纸质处方、电子处方和病区用药医嘱单。

（二）处方审核形式

1. 人工审核　药师对处方的合法性、规范性、适宜性各项内容进行逐一审核。

2. 信息系统辅助审核　医疗机构信息系统配置合理用药软件，合理用药软件对处方进行初步审核，对合理用药软件不能审核的部分以及合理用药软件筛选出的不合理处方，由药师进行人工审核或复核。

（三）处方审核依据

包括药品说明书、国家药品管理相关法律法规和规范性文件、国家处方集、国家卫生主管部门发布的临床诊疗规范和指南、临床路径等。

（四）处方审核流程

1. 接收待审核处方，对处方进行合法性、规范性、适宜性审核；

2. 若经审核判定为合理处方，药师在处方上进行手写签名、电子签名或签章，处方经药师签名或签章后进入收费和调配环节；

3. 若经审核判定为不合理处方，药师联系处方医师，建议其修改或者重新开具处方，经处方医师修改或重新开具的处方再次进入处方审核流程。若处方医师不同意修改或重新开具处方，药师应当做好记录，对于严重不合理用药或者用药错误，拒绝审核通过，并上报医务部门。审方药师判定为合理处方，核对药品无误后发药并指导患者用药，包括用药方法、时间、剂量、注意事项等。对于无法准确判断合理性的处方，处方审核药师应与处方医师沟通联系，必要时向上级药师、处方科室上级医师或处方审核专家组寻求技术支持（图4-3-1）。

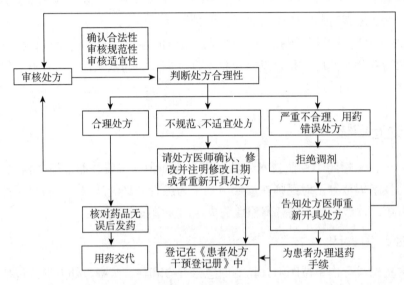

图 4-3-1　处方审核流程

四、用药咨询

用药咨询是指药师利用药学专业知识和工具向患者、患者家属、医务人员以及公众提供药物信息，宣传合理用药知识，交流与用药相关问题的过程。

1. 用药咨询服务对象　包括患者、患者家属、医务人员和公众等。

2. 用药咨询的方式　可包括面对面咨询、电话咨询和互联网咨询。

3. 用药咨询内容　可包括药品的名称、用法用量、疗效、用药注意事项、药物间相互作用、贮存方法、药品不良反应识别及处置，以及特殊剂型指导、患者用药教育和疾病的预防等。

4. 用药咨询服务流程　包括接待咨询者、询问咨询者需求、采集用药史及相关病史、分析评估、及时回答咨询者问题。用药咨询药师在提供用药咨询服务时，应及时对相关信息进行记录，记录内容包括咨询者姓名、性别、出生年月日、药品名称、咨询问题、解答内容以及参考依据等。

五、药物重整

药物重整是指比较患者目前正在应用的所有药物方案与药物医嘱是否一致的过程。其详细定义包括在患者药物治疗的每一个不同阶段（入院、转科或出院时），药师通过与患者沟通或复核，了解在医疗交接前后的整体用药情况是否一致，与医疗团队一起对不适当的用药进行调整，并做详细全面的记录，来预防医疗过程中的药物不良事件，保证患者用药安全的过程。

（一）重整实施过程

药物重整应贯穿整个医疗过程，尤其是在医疗团队发生改变时（入院、转科或出院）必须进行药物重整。所有用药的调整，须与医师充分沟通，通过与患者或患者家属面谈、电话询问负责患者用药的家属或监护人、查阅患者既往病历及处方信息等方式采集既往用药史。既往用药史的内容应包括目前正在使用药物及既往使用过的与疾病密切相关药物（包括处方药、非处方药、中成药/中草药以及疫苗等）和保健品的名称、剂型和规格、用法用量、用药起止时间、停药原因、依从性等。还应采集药物及食物过敏史相关信息，根据既往用药史建立药物重整记录。

（二）药物重整应重点关注的内容

1. 核查用药适应证及是否存在重复用药问题。
2. 核查用法用量是否正确。
3. 关注特殊剂型/装置药物，给药途径是否恰当。
4. 关注需要根据肝肾功能调整剂量的药物，必要时进行剂量调整。
5. 关注存在潜在相互作用、可能发生不良反应的药物，必要时调整药物治疗方案。
6. 关注症状缓解药物，这些药物是药物重整的重点，明确此类药物是否需要长期使用。
7. 关注特殊人群用药，如高龄老年人、儿童、妊娠期与哺乳期妇女、肝肾功能不全者、精神疾病患者等，综合考虑患者药物治疗的安全性、有效性、适宜性及依从性。
8. 核查拟行特殊检查或医疗操作前是否需要临时停用某些药物，检查或操作结束后，需评估是否续用药物。
9. 关注静脉药物及有明确疗程的药物是否继续使用。

六、用药教育

用药教育，是指对患者进行合理用药指导，为患者普及合理用药知识，目的是增强患者用药知识，预防药品不良反应的发生，提高患者用药依从性，并降低用药错误的发生率。

（一）用药教育的步骤

1. 向患者自我介绍，说明此次教育的目的和预期时间。

2. 收集患者疾病史、用药史、文化程度等信息，根据初步沟通确定用药教育的方式（口头或书面），充分考虑患者的特殊情况，如视力、听力、语言不通等。

3. 评估患者对自身健康问题和用药情况的了解及期望、正确使用药物的能力以及对治疗的态度。

4. 通过开放式询问的方式，了解患者对用药目的、药物服用方法、服用剂量、服药疗程、用药注意事项、常见不良反应等方面的掌握程度；结合患者的现有用药知识基础，制定个体化用药教育方案。

5. 采取一种或多种适合个体患者的教育方式进行用药教育，使患者充分了解药物治疗的重要性和药品的正确使用方式。

6. 用药教育结束前需验证患者对药物使用的知识和掌握程度，请患者复述用药教育重点内容，根据患者的接受效果调整用药教育方式，并再次进行用药教育直至患者完全掌握。

7. 如实记录用药教育记录。

（二）用药教育的内容

1. 药物（或药物装置）的通用名、商品名或其他常用名称，以及药物的治疗分类、用途及预期效果。

2. 药物的预计起效时间及未起效时的应对措施。

3. 药物剂型、给药途径、剂量、用药时间和疗程。

4. 药物的特殊剂型、特殊装置、特殊配制方法的用药说明，可依据患者的生活方式或环境进行相应的调整。

5. 用药期间应监测的症状体征及检验指标，解释药物可能对相关临床检验结果的干扰以及对排泄物颜色造成的改变。

6. 可能出现的常见和严重的不良反应，可采取的预防措施及发生不良反应后的应急措施；发生用药错误（如漏服药物）时可能产生的结果，以及应对措施。

7. 潜在的药物–药物、药物–食物/保健品、药物–疾病及药物–环境的相互作用或禁忌。

8. 药物的适宜贮存条件，过期药或废弃装置的适当处理。

9. 如何做好用药记录和自我监测，以及如何及时联系药师。

七、药学查房

药学查房，是指以临床药师为主体，在病区内对患者开展以安全、合理、有效用药为目的的查房过程。包括药师独立查房和药师与医师、护士医疗团队的联合查房。

（一）药学查房的环境与对象

1. 临床药师应在选定专业的临床科室开展药学查房。

2. 临床药师宜对提请药学会诊的患者开展药学查房。

3. 药学常规查房的开展场所应为病床旁。

（二）查房准备

1. 明确药学查房的患者数量及预期的查房时间。

2. 获取并熟悉患者的基本情况，尤其是重点监护患者如病危、病重、病情复杂及新入院患者等，内容包括但不限于患者姓名、性别、年龄、生命体征、现病史、基础疾病、既往史、既往用药史、过敏史、家族史、个人史、婚育史、入院诊断、辅助检查结果、治疗方案及疾病进展等情况。

3. 在熟悉患者资料过程中，对于存在疑问或着重了解的部分应做好相应记录。

4. 对新入院患者院外使用药物进行药物重整，整理患者此次入院的初始治疗方案，对重点药物如抗菌药物、糖皮质激素、抗肿瘤药物及各专科相关重点药物等进行重点监护。

5. 从药物的有效性、安全性、经济性和适宜性等方面对初始治疗方案进行用药合理性分析，记录和干预不合理医嘱。

（1）用药有效性分析　应包括但不限于药物适应证、用法用量、给药途径和疗程等。

（2）用药安全性分析　包括但不限于防治药物不良反应、药物相互作用评估等。

（3）用药经济性分析　包括但不限于医疗保险和患者承受能力等。

（4）用药适宜性分析　包括但不限于皮试结果、药品规格和重复用药等。

6. 对在院患者的医嘱分析应考虑疾病进展、辅助检查结果和治疗方案调整等，特别是可能影响用药的诊断修订、实验室检查结果更新（如肝脏和肾脏功能变化等）、合并用药改变和重要医嘱增减等变化情况。通过合理用药分析提炼出药学问诊的内容、患者教育的要点和药学查房的思路与内容等。

7. 新入院患者查房记录表格内容应包括但不限于患者基本情况、患者诊断、实验室检查结果、院外医嘱重整、初始治疗方案、用药有效性、安全性、经济性和适宜性分析、不合理用药干预、药学问诊内容、依从性评价、患者教育、问题及患者反馈等。在院患者查房记录表格内容应包括但不限于患者基本情况、患者诊断、修正诊断、实验室检查结果更新、治疗方案调整、调整后方案、用药有效性、安全性、经济性和适宜性分析、不合理用药干预、药学问诊内容、患者教育、问题及患者反馈等。

（三）查房过程

1. 对患者进行初次查房时，应进行简单的自我介绍，告知患者临床药师身份和临床药师在住院期间能够提供的药学服务。告知患者药学查房的主要目的在于宣教与用药相关的注意事项，促进药物的合理应用。

2. 药学问诊的主要内容包含患者整个诊疗过程中的所有疾病和药物相关信息，评估患者药物治疗的获益和风险，获取患者治疗需求，为药学监护的制定和实施提供基础信息和客观证据。

3. 重点关注患者用药问题，核实患者是否按要求用药、用药后的反应、是否有不适情况、嗜好、生活方式等信息，以便有针对性地进行用药教育，指导患者正确使用治疗药物，为患者制定药学监护计划。

4. 对刚入院患者，药师应与患者或家属积极进行交流，询问患者此次入院治疗目的，既往所患疾病及用药情况，药物及食物过敏史，药物不良反应及处置史等基本信息。对患者既往用药，应详细询问药品名称、药品规格、给药途径、剂量、疗程、疗效等。如患者存在药物过敏史，应询问过敏药物名称、过敏症状、体征、转归等。

5. 对诊治过程中的患者，应询问患者对自身疾病、服用药物的知晓情况，是否遵医嘱用药。询问患者使用药物后的症状、体征改善情况，是否有新发症状，判断患者目前药物治疗的临床疗效。制定监护计划，包括患者指标的变化、不良反应的观察与判断、给药方案的变化、是否需要给药方案调整等。

6. 患者用药教育的方式包括语言教育、书面教育、实物演示教育等。用药教育的内容包括普适性的用药教育、特殊剂型的用药教育、特殊人群的用药教育及特殊药物的用药教育等。用药教育的具体内容应包括药品名称（商品名及通用名）、药品规格、药品性状、用药原因、用法与用量、服药时间（空腹/餐时/餐后等）和服药方法（吞服、嚼服等）、常见不良反应、注意事项（包括药物–药物、药物–食物相互作用）、漏服处理策略及贮藏方式等，还包括饮食、生活方式、疾病相关指标（血压、血脂、血糖等）的监测及复诊等。用药教育后，宜向患者发放用药教育材料，巩固用药教育成果。

7. 临床药师根据药学评估结果，整理出患者用药问题，查找文献，分析问题，给出问题解决方案及建议，及时与医生、护士及患者沟通。

八、用药监护

用药监护，是指医疗机构药师应用药学专业知识向住院患者提供直接的、负责任的、与药物使用相关的监护，以期提高药物治疗的安全性、有效性与经济性。

分级用药监护，是指患者在住院期间，药师根据患者的病理生理状态、疾病特点和用药情况进行评定从而确定的监护级别。

监护过程：

1. 住院患者用药监护应贯穿于患者药物治疗的全过程，从患者进入病区接诊开始，至转出或离院为止。如患者有转科情况，再次转回病区后，应重新评估并实施患者监护，至再次转出或离院为止。

2. 根据患者所接受的治疗药物情况、患者特殊的病理生理状态等确定监护对象。药师应依据用药监护分级标准对患者所需的用药监护服务进行分级。对于特殊专科患者，如肿瘤、血液、儿科等，可根据上述标准酌情调整。

3. 针对患者的用药监护分级，可参照药物监测分级开展不同级别的用药监护工作。药师可利用药物基因检测、治疗药物监测等手段，结合药动学和药效学情况，制定个体化用药治疗方案，对患者实行用药监护。

4. 建立规范的患者用药监护记录表，如实记录患者住院期间的药物治疗情况。

5. 针对不适宜的药物治疗，药师应及时将具体建议、参考依据及医师和（或）护士反馈结果等内容进行记录。

九、居家药学服务

居家药学服务，是指医疗机构为患者居家药物治疗提供个体化、全程、连续的药学服务和健康知识普及，开展用药评估、用药教育，帮助患者提高用药依从性，保障药品贮存和安全、合理使用，进而改善治疗结果。药师可以依据需求准备分药盒、药物教具（如胰岛素笔、吸入制剂装置等）、测量仪器（如血糖仪、血压计、体重秤、峰流速仪、皮尺等器具）、管理患者慢性疾病的表格（如峰流速记录表）等物品。

（一）服务过程

居家药学服务对象主要包括签约家庭医生服务的居民，以及易发生药物相关问题的重点服务人群。

（二）居家药学服务具体内容

包括但并不限于以下内容：

1. **药物重整、药物治疗管理**　对于高诊次患者，以及用药种数多的居民，药师可提供药物重整和药物治疗管理服务，提出用药相关建议，并与患者的主治医生或其他专科医生进行沟通协商，最终确定患者的新用药治疗方案。由药师对患者进行全面的用药指导和用药教育。

2. **用药咨询**　当患者对自己的药物有疑问或者担忧时，药师可提供用药咨询服务。

3. **用药教育**　对于特殊患者、特殊药物，药师可提供用药教育服务。特殊患者包括但不限于近期出现药物治疗重要变化（如出院刚回到家中）、意识不清或不能吞咽完整药物的患者；特殊药物包括但不限于高风险药物（如抗凝药、胰岛素、治疗窗窄的药物）、装置复杂的药物（如吸入制剂等）。

4. **科普宣教**　为居家患者进行科普宣传，选择个性化的科普宣教方式，使用通俗易懂的语言将正确的用药信息传播给患者，指导患者用药安全、有效、经济和适宜。

5. **清理家庭药箱**　药师定期或不定期检查居民家中药品的有效期、性状，对居民进行药品存放指导和过期或变质药品回收服务指导等。

（三）居家药学服务一般流程

1. 在基层医疗机构或居民家中提供服务，药师应着工作服、佩戴胸牌，按预约时间提供服务。

2. 按照制定的计划对居民进行药学服务。

3. 如需对患者处方药物进行调整，药师应先和家庭医生沟通，并将调整建议以书面形式交给家庭医生参考，由医生进行处方更改。

4. 对于服务内容、药物清单等内容进行记录。

5. 发现的药物相关问题与居民交代或与医生沟通的情况应记录在干预记录表中。

6. 在服务完成后应请服务对象或监护人对服务完成情况进行确认签字。

7. 如需要再次进行服务，药师应与居民约定下次服务时间，并在随访表上记录患者实验室指标的改变情况、下次随访时间和随访内容。

（四）居家药学服务可参考的依据

包括：药品说明书、国家药品管理相关法律法规和规范性文件、国家处方集、临床诊疗规范和指南、临床路径等。对于服务内容、服务过程中发现的问题以及药师和居民、医师沟通的结果应做好记录，相关记录应可溯源。

十、急诊药学服务

急诊药学是药学服务的一个分支，主要执行单位是医院的急诊药房，工作任务由急诊药房的急诊药师来承担，急诊药学服务时间主要是下班后和夜间。急诊药学就是急诊与药学的共同体，一是体现急，二是围绕药来进行相关医疗服务的事宜。

（一）急诊药学服务特点

医务人员被动的迎接每例就诊病人，面对的是急救、中毒、外伤、交通事故、重症、转院来诊和婴幼儿及老弱病人，而突发事件中的病人数量多、病情急、情绪不稳定等。

（二）急诊药学服务内容

1. 需合理备药，确保急救药品充足。设置急救药品专区，便于急救时易于调配。药师熟悉《急诊药房常备抢救用药品目录》《反恐卫生应急药品储备目录》等有关急救药品目录，熟练掌握并应用"库存预警"系统，做好每日请领药品工作。定期对急救药品数量及有效期进行盘点，做到实物与库存相符，保证药品质量。

2. 充分审查医嘱中药物的相互作用、配伍禁忌、药物的用法用量、给药途径，发现不合理用药，立即联系医师，提出合理用药建议，做到用药前干预，最大限度地保证用药安全。

3. 开展用药咨询，准确提供药学信息。对于特别需要注意和新进的药品，药师首先仔细阅读说明书，及时反馈信息给医师或提供相关资料。对于窗口患者咨询的用药问题给予认真仔细地解答，并为患者解除用药方面的心理障碍。

4. 重视过敏反应，药师审核处方时要关注以下信息：①药品说明书明确要求进行皮试的药品；②过敏体质病人；③病人有青霉素类或头孢类药物过敏史或皮试阳性史；④处方中若药物剂量过大，与医生沟通。

Appendix

Appendix 1 The Conversion Ratio of Drug Dosage between Animals

Animal	K Value	Weight Range (kg)	Conversion Factor mg/kg–mg/m^2	The Ratio of Body Surface Area per Body Weight
Mouse	9.1	0.018~0.024	3	1.0(0.02kg)
Rat	9.1	0.05~0.25	6	0.47(0.20kg)
Guinea Pig	9.8	0.30~0.60	8	0.40(0.40kg)
Rabbit	10.1	1.50~2.50	12	0.24(2.0kg)
Cat	9.9	2.00~3.00	14	0.22(2.5kg)
Dog	11.2	5.00~15.0	19	0.16(10.0kg)
Monkey	11.8	2.00~4.00	12	0.24(3.0kg)
Human	10.6	40.0~60.0	36	0.08(50.0kg)

Appendix 2 Common Administration Volume on Lab Animals

Animal	Route of Administration	Abbreviation	Suitable Administration Volume
Mouse	Gavage	i.g.	0.1~0.3 ml/10g
	Subcutaneous	s.c.	0.05~0.2 ml/10g
	Intraperitoneal	i.p.	0.1~0.3 ml/10g
	Intramuscular	i.m.	0.02~0.05 ml/10g
	Tail vein	i.v.	0.1~0.2 ml/10g
Rat	Gavage	i.g.	1~3 ml/100g
	Subcutaneous	s.c.	0.5~1 ml/100g
	Intraperitoneal	i.p.	0.5~1 ml/100g
	Intramuscular	i.m.	0.1~0.2 ml/100g
Rabbit	Gavage	i.g.	5~20 ml/kg
	Subcutaneous	s.c.	0.5~1 ml/kg
	Intraperitoneal	i.p.	1~5 ml/kg
	Intramuscular	i.m.	0.5~1 ml/kg
	Ear vein	i.v.	0.2~2 ml/kg

Appendix 3　Common Dosage of Anaesthetics for Injection

Drug and Concentration	Animal	Route of Administration	Dosage (mg/kg)	Duration (h)
Sodium Pentobarbital (30g/L)	Dog	*i.v.* , *i.p.*	30~35	1~4
	Cat, Rabbit and Rat	*i.p.*	40	1~4
Sodium Thiopental (50g/L)	Dog	*i.v.*	15~50	1/4~1/2
	Rabbit	*i.v.*	15~80	1/4~1/2
	Cat	*i.p.*	25~80	1/2~1
	Rat	*i.p.*	50	1/2~1
Uratan (200g/L)	Rabbit	*i.v.*	1000	2~4
	Rat	*i.p.*	1000~1500	2~4
	Cat	*i.p.*	1000	2~4
Chloralose (20g/L)	Dog, Rabbit	*i.v.*	60~100	5~6
	Rat	*i.p.*	50~80	5~6
	Cat	*i.m.*	34	5~6

Note: Formulate anaesthetics for injection with distilled water or normal saline. Sodium thiopental is unstable, therefore prepare it just before the injection.

Appendix 4　Physiological Constants of Common Lab Animals

Animal	Dog	Cat	Rabbit	Guinea Pig	Rat	Mouse
Weight(kg)	5~15	2~3	1.5~2.5	0.3~0.6	0.1~0.2	0.018~0.025
Average Body Temperature(℃)	38.5	38.5	39.0	39.5	38.0	37.4
Breath Rate(Time/ Minute)	20~30	25~50	55~90	100~150	100~150	126~136
Heart Rate(Time/ Minute)	100~200	120~180	150~220	180~250	250~400	400~600
Blood Pressure(kPa)	16.7/6.7	17.3/10	14/10	10.7	14.7	15.3
Full Blood Volume(ml/100g)	7.8	7.2	7.2	5.8	6.0	7.8
Concentration of Haemoglobin(mg/L)	110~180	70~150	80~150	110~165	120~175	100~190

Continued Table

Animal	Dog	Cat	Rabbit	Guinea Pig	Rat	Mouse
Concentration of platelet(10^4/mm^3)	10~60	10~50	38~52	68~87	50~100	60~110

Appendix 5 Common Physiological Solutions Unit（g/L）

Drug	NormaL Saline	Tyrode	Krebs	Riger-Locke	Krebs-Hense Leit	Riger
NaCl	9.0	8.0	6.60	9.0	6.92	7.0
KCl		0.2	0.35	0.2	0.35	0.14
MgCl$_2$		0.1				
CaCl$_2$		0.2	0.28	0.2	0.28	0.12
NaH$_2$PO$_4$		0.05				
KH$_2$PO$_4$			0.16		0.16	
NaHCO$_3$		1.0	2.1	0.3	2.1	0.2
MgSO$_4$			0.29		0.29	
Glucose		1.0	2.0	1.0	2.0	1.0
Ventilation		Air	O$_2$+5%CO$_2$	O$_2$	O$_2$+5%CO$_2$	
Application	Small Amount *i.v* to Mammals	Mammal Intestinal Muscle	Various Tissues of Mammals and Birds	Mammal Heart	Isolated Guinea Pig Trachea, etc.	Frog Organs

Instruction

1. The composition, content and application of each solution in the table are different but similar.

2. Any solution containing NaHCO$_3$, NaH$_2$PO$_4$ or CaCl$_2$ should be dissolved separately, and then added to other fully dissolved and diluted ingredients, to prevent precipitation.

3. Add glucose just before use to prevent deterioration.

Appendix 6 Common Latin Abbreviations

Abbreviation	Latin	English
1. Dose Form		
caps.	capsula	Capsule

Continued Table

Abbreviation	Latin	English
inj.	injection	Injection
neb.	nebula	Spray
naristtill.	naristilla	Collunarium Nasal drop
ocul.	oculentum	Eye Ointmert
supp.	suppositorium	Suppository
tab.	tabella	Tablet
2. Dose Unit		
s.s.	semisse	Semi−dose, in half
gtt.	guttae	Prop
i.u. or *U*	international unit	International unit
q.s.	quantum satis	Proper quantities
D.t.d.	Da(dentur) tales doses	Equal amounts
3. Routes of Administration		
i.h.	injectio hypodermica	Subcutaneous injection
i.m.	injectio muscularis	Intramuscular injection
i.v.	injectio venosa	Intravenous injection
i.v.gtt.	injectio venosa gutta	Drip phleboclysis
p.o.	per os	Orally
p.r.	per rectum	Per rectum
pro o.	pro oculis	Ophthalmic use
pro aur.	pro auribus	Aural use
pro nar.	pro naribus	Nasal use
us.ext.	usum externum	External use
4. Dose Frequency		
b.i.d.	bis in die	Twice daily
q.d.	quaque die	Once daily
q.i.d.	quarter in die	Four times daily
q.o.d.	quaque omni die	Once every other day
q.h.	quaque hora	Once every an hour
q.4h.	quaque quarta hora	Once every four hours
q.m.	quaque mane	Once every morning
q.n.	quaque nocte	Once every night
t.i.d.	ter in die	Three times daily

Appendix 7 Implementation Regulations for Pharmacy Service Etiquette

According to industry and job features, pharmacy service etiquette generally includes the following requirements:

1. The appearance should be dignified and tidy

1.1 Hair: hair should be washed and combed frequently. Male hair should not be too long, and the hairstyle should be suitable for work and social places.

1.2 Hands: the nail should not be too long and not be painted with nail polish. Personnel in the preparation room should cut the nails short according to regulations and should not wear the ring.

1.3 Beard: male should not have a beard and should develop the habit of daily shaving.

1.4 Mouth: keep clean, and do not chew gum during working hours. Do not drink alcohol or eat food with peculiar smell before work.

1.5 Make-Up: it is recommended for ladies to wear light make-up. The makeup should give people a fresh, elegant and natural image. Heavy make-up are not suitable in the workplace. Besides, earrings and strong fragrance perfume should not be worn.

2. Dress up for the shift, wear a badge, and be neat and tidy

2.1 Dress: work clothes should be changed and washed regularly. The time for changing long or short-sleeved work clothes each year is uniformly stipulated by the institution due to the season. Men's short-sleeved work clothes must be worn with a vest or short-sleeved shirt.

2.2 Badge: it should be worn as required, and surface of the badge should be kept clean. Do not let the back of it face outwards.

2.3 Shirts: collar and cuffs of the shirt should not be dirty and should be ironed flat.

2.4 Tie: Men are advised to wear a tie. The tie should be plain colour and should not be defaced, slanted or loose.

2.5 Footwear: keep clean and no slipper during the shift.

3. Medical staff should maintain elegant postures and movements

3.1 Standing: keep heels on the ground with toes slightly outward, the back and chest naturally straight, head slightly downward and arms naturally drop without shrugging the shoulder. Besides, the gravity centre of the body should be between feet. Do not cross hands on the chest.

3.2 Sitting: the sitting posture should be upright with legs parallel. When move the chair, put the chair in the position first, then sit.

3.3 Dispensing Drugs: be gentle when distribute medicines. Keep the medicine neat with words facing to the patient. Must not throw drugs to the patient.

4. Answer and dial the phone quickly, correctly and politely

4.1 When hear the phone ringing, answer it as quickly as possible, however it is strictly prohibited to answer the phone when distribute the prescription. When talking, you should greet first, and inform the hospital and department. Listen carefully and write down main points. If not hear clearly, tell the other party in time. Say goodbye politely at the end of the call, and wait until the other party cuts off the phone, afterwards hang off the phone.

4.2 The call should be concise, and no chatting on the phone. No private call without special circumstance.

4.3 For the call that can not be handled, tell the other party to make another call or immediately hand the call to someone who can handle it.

5. Receiving patients with civilised language, friendly attitude, and cordial and natural manner

5.1 Patients should be treated equally. Must not judge any people on their appearance.

5.2 All verbal actions should be based on the respect for patients. Be polite and call the patient with an accurate and appropriate appellation. If the name on the prescription is clear, call the name naturally and kindly. Do not use imperative and untitled sentences that may make people feel disrespectful.

5.3 Use civilised words, such as 'please', 'sorry', and 'thank you'. When talk to the patient, look directly at them.

5.4 Fully understand the patient. If there's problem with the prescription or the patient's procedure of taking drugs, clearly but euphemistically inform the patient, along with the method and procedure for corrections.

5.5 Provide convenience to patients as much as possible, and help solve problem. Do not shirk responsibility.

6. Answer patients' questions patiently and enthusiastically

6.1 Answer the patient's questions patiently and enthusiastically on any occasion in the hospital. Do not say 'I don't know' or 'I'm not sure'. If you really don't know how to answer the patient's question, you should kindly inform the patient with relevant departments.

6.2 While meeting patients asking for directions, patiently and enthusiastically indicate the route, supplemented by appropriate gestures when necessary. In the event of elderly patients who are physically weak or disabled, lead the way if possible.

7. Other etiquette

Before entering the room, gently knock on the door first, then enter after hearing the answer. Afterwards, turn back and close the door, not vigorously. After entering the room, if the other is talking, wait for a while and don't interrupt. However, when in a hurry, you should take advantage of the opportunity and boldly say 'sorry, I have to interrupt your conversation'.

When walk in aisles and corridors, take light steps and not talk loudly, let alone singing or whistling. While encountering the elderly or patients, be courteous and do not rush. When in a hurry, you should say 'sorry' first.

While submitting objects, such as business cards, documents, etc., keep them face up. If it is a pen, point the pen tip towards yourself. When submiting sharp tools, such as knives or scissors, must be pointed towards you.

附　录

附录一　常用动物间剂量换算参数

动物	K 值	体重范围（kg）	转换因子 / mg/kg–mg/m²	每 kg 体重占体表面积比值
小鼠	9.1	0.018~0.024	3	1.0（0.02kg）
大鼠	9.1	0.05~0.25	6	0.47（0.20kg）
豚鼠	9.8	0.30~0.60	8	0.40（0.40kg）
兔	10.1	1.50~2.50	12	0.24（2.0kg）
猫	9.9	2.00~3.00	14	0.22（2.5kg）
狗	11.2	5.00~15.0	19	0.16（10.0kg）
猴	11.8	2.00~4.00	12	0.24（3.0kg）
人	10.6	40.0~60.0	36	0.08（50.0kg）

附录二　常用实验动物给药容量

动物	给药途径	英文（拉丁）缩写	适宜给药容量
小鼠	灌胃	*i.g.*	0.1~0.3 ml/10g
	皮下注射	*s.c.*	0.05~0.2 ml/10g
	腹腔注射	*i.p.*	0.1~0.3 ml/10g
	肌肉注射	*i.m.*	0.02~0.05 ml/10g
	尾静脉注射	*i.v.*	0.1~0.2 ml/10g
大鼠	灌胃	*i.g.*	1~3 ml/100g
	皮下注射	*s.c.*	0.5~1 ml/100g
	腹腔注射	*i.p.*	0.5~1 ml/100g
	肌肉注射	*i.m.*	0.1~0.2 ml/100g

续表

动物	给药途径	英文（拉丁）缩写	适宜给药容量
家兔	灌胃	*i.g.*	5~20 ml/kg
	皮下注射	*s.c.*	0.5~1 ml/kg
	腹腔注射	*i.p.*	1~5 ml/kg
	肌肉注射	*i.m.*	0.5~1 ml/kg
	耳缘静脉注射	*i.v.*	0.2~2 ml/kg

附录三　常用注射麻醉药物用量

药物及浓度	动物	给药途径	剂量 /（mg/kg）	维持时间 /（小时）
戊巴比妥钠 （30g/L）	狗	*i.v., i.p.*	30~35	1~4
	猫、兔、大鼠	*i.p.*	40	1~4
硫喷妥钠 （50g/L）	狗	*i.v.*	15~50	1/4~1/2
	兔	*i.v.*	15~80	1/4~1/2
	猫	*i.p.*	25~80	1/2~1
	大鼠	*i.p.*	50	1/2~1
乌拉坦 （200g/L）	兔	*i.v.*	1000	2~4
	大鼠	*i.p.*	1000~1500	2~4
	猫	*i.p.*	1000	2~4
氯醛糖 （20g/L）	狗、兔	*i.v.*	60~100	5~6
	大鼠	*i.p.*	50~80	5~6
	猫	*i.m.*	34	5~6

注意事项：配制注射用麻醉剂，可用蒸馏水或生理盐水。硫喷妥钠溶液不稳定，应现用现配。

附录四　常用实验动物生理常数值

动物种类	狗	猫	兔	豚鼠	大鼠	小鼠
适用体重（kg）	5~15	2~3	1.5~2.5	0.3~0.6	0.1~0.2	0.018~0.025
平均体温（℃）	38.5	38.5	39.0	39.5	38.0	37.4
呼吸频率（次/分）	20~30	25~50	55~90	100~150	100~150	126~136
心率（次/分）	100~200	120~180	150~220	180~250	250~400	400~600
血压（kPa）	16.7/6.7	17.3/10	14/10	10.7	14.7	15.3
血量（ml/100g）	7.8	7.2	7.2	5.8	6.0	7.8

续表

动物种类	狗	猫	兔	豚鼠	大鼠	小鼠
血红蛋白（mg/L）	110~180	70~150	80~150	110~165	120~175	100~190
血小板（万/mm^3）	10~60	10~50	38~52	68~87	50~100	60~110

附录五　常用生理溶液

单位（g/L）

药品	生理盐水	台氏液	克氏液	任洛氏液	克亨氏液	任氏液
NaCl	9.0	8.0	6.60	9.0	6.92	7.0
KCl		0.2	0.35	0.2	0.35	0.14
MgCl$_2$		0.1				
CaCl$_2$		0.2	0.28	0.2	0.28	0.12
NaH$_2$PO$_4$		0.05				
KH$_2$PO$_4$			0.16		0.16	
NaHCO$_3$		1.0	2.1	0.3	2.1	0.2
MgSO$_4$			0.29		0.29	
GLucose		1.0	2.0	1.0	2.0	1.0
通气		空气	O$_2$+5%CO$_2$	O$_2$	O$_2$+5%CO$_2$	
用途	哺乳类小量	哺乳类肠肌	哺乳类及鸟类各种组织	哺乳类心脏	豚鼠离体气管等	蛙类器官

说明：1.表中各溶液成分、含量和用途各家不一，但大同小异。

2.凡溶液中含有NaHCO$_3$、NaH$_2$PO$_4$或CaCl$_2$，应先分别溶解，然后加入其他已充分溶解稀释的成分中，以防止产生沉淀。

3.葡萄糖临用前加入，以防变质。

附录六　常用拉丁文缩写词

缩写词	原文（Latin）	中文（Chinese）
1. 药物制剂		
caps.	capsula	胶囊
inj.	injection	注射剂
neb.	nebula	喷雾剂
naristtill.	naristilla	滴鼻剂
ocul.	oculentum	眼膏剂
supp.	suppositorium	栓剂
tab.	tabella	片剂

续表

缩写词	原文（Latin）	中文（Chinese）
2. 剂量单位		
s.s.	semisse	一半
gtt.	guttae	滴
i.u. 或 *U*	international unit	国际单位
q.s.	quantum satis	适量
D.t.d.	Da(dentur) tales doses	给予同量
3. 给药途径		
i.h.	injectio hypodermica	皮下注射
i.m.	injectio muscularis	肌肉注射
i.v.	injectio venosa	静脉注射
i.v.gtt.	injectio venosa gutta	静脉滴注
p.o.	per os	口服
p.r.	per rectum	直肠给药，灌肠
pro o.	pro oculis	眼用
pro aur.	pro auribus	耳用
pro nar.	pro naribus	鼻用
us.ext.	usum externum	外用
4. 给药次数		
b.i.d.	bis in die	每日二次
q.d.	quaque die	每日一次
q.i.d.	quarter in die	每日四次
q.o.d.	quaque omni die	隔日一次
q.h.	quaque hora	每小时一次
q.4h.	quaque quarta hora	每四小时一次
q.m.	quaque mane	每晨一次
q.n.	quaque nocte	每晚一次
t.i.d.	ter in die	每日三次

附录七　药学工作服务礼仪执行条例

根据行业和工作特点，药学服务礼仪大致包括以下一些要求：

第一条：仪表端庄、整洁

（1）头发：头发要经常清洗和梳理。男性头发不宜太长，发型应适合工作和社交场所的要求。

（2）手部：指甲不能太长，不得涂指甲油；制剂室人员应按规定剪指甲并不得佩戴戒指。

（3）胡子：男性不宜留胡须，应养成每日剃须的习惯。

（4）口腔：应保持清洁，工作时间不能咀嚼口香糖；上班前不能喝酒或吃有异味的食品。

（5）化妆：提倡女士化淡妆。化妆应给人清新、淡雅和自然的形象，工作场合不宜化浓妆，不宜配戴耳环和使用香味浓烈的香水。

第二条：着装上岗，佩戴胸卡，服装整洁

（1）着装：工作服定期换洗。每年更换长、短袖工作服时间由单位根据季节变化统一规定；男士短袖工作服内须着背心或短袖衫。

（2）胸卡：应按规定佩戴，胸卡表面应保持清洁，不得背面向外。

（3）衬衫：衬衫领口与袖口不得污秽，最好熨烫平整。

（4）领带：提倡男士佩戴领带，领带以素色较为适宜，不得有污损或歪斜松弛。

（5）鞋袜：保持清洁，工作时间不得穿拖鞋。

第三条：工作人员应保持优雅的姿势和动作

（1）站姿：两脚跟着地，脚尖微向外，腰背胸膛自然挺直，头微向下，两臂自然下垂，不耸肩，身体重心在两脚中间。不得把手交叉抱在胸前。

（2）坐姿：坐姿应端正，双腿平行放好，要移动椅子时，应先把椅子放好位置，然后再坐。

（3）发药：发放药品时，动作宜轻柔，应将药品轻轻摆放整齐，正面向上、文字正向对方；切不可将药品随意丢给患者甚至扔向对方。

第四条：迅速、正确、礼貌地接、打电话

（1）听到电话铃响，应尽可能快地接听（正在配方发药时，严禁接听电话）。通话时应先问候"您好"，并自报医院和科室。对方讲述要认真仔细听，并记下要点。未听清时，及时告诉对方，结束时礼貌道别，待对方切断电话，自己再放话筒。

（2）通话应简明扼要，不得在电话中聊天。无特殊情况不得接打私人电话。

（3）对自己不能处理的电话内容，可告知对方拨打其他电话或马上将电话交给能够处理的人。

第五条：语言文明、态度和蔼、亲切自然地接待病人

（1）对待患者应一视同仁，不得以貌取人。

（2）一切言语行动均应以尊重患者为出发点，做到礼貌、客气，称谓需准确、恰当，处方上姓名清楚的可自然亲切地直呼姓名。禁止使用让人感觉不尊重的命令式和无称谓的语句。

（3）必须使用"您""请""对不起""谢谢"等文明用语。与患者对话时，必须直视对方。

（4）应充分理解和体谅患者，患者取药时，如处方或患者的取药程序有问题，应明确但委婉地向患者指出，并告知改正的方法和程序。

（5）尽可能地为患者提供方便，帮助解决问题，不推卸责任，不推诿病人。

第六条：热情耐心地回答患者的问题

（1）在医院内的任何场合，都要热情耐心地回答患者的问题，不允许说"不知道"、"不清楚"。如果患者提出的问题自己确实不了解，应善意地提示患者到相关的部门去询问。

（2）遇到患者问路，应热情耐心地为患者指明，需要时辅以适当的手势。如遇年迈体衰或有残疾的患者，应尽可能亲自为患者引路。

第七条：其他礼仪

进入房间，要先轻轻敲门，听到应答后再进入。进入后，回手关门，不能大力、粗暴。进入房间后，如对方正在讲话，要稍等静候，不要中途插话，但如有急事要看准机会大胆说话，并要先说"对不起，打断你们的谈话了。"在通道、走廊上走路，要放轻脚步，不能边走边大声说话，更不能唱歌或吹口哨等。遇到长者或患者要礼让，不能抢行；遇有急事需要抢行时，应说"对不起"。递交物件时（如名片、文件等），要正面向上、文字朝着对方递上；如果是笔，要把笔尖向着自己；刀子或剪刀等利器，应把刀尖向着自己。